MULTIPLE SCLEROSIS
SOURCEBOOK
THIRD EDITION

Health Reference Series

MULTIPLE SCLEROSIS
SOURCEBOOK

THIRD EDITION

Provides Basic Consumer Health Information about Multiple Sclerosis and Related Conditions, including Autoimmune Diseases, Chronic Inflammatory Demyelinating Polyneuropathy, Neuromyelitis Optica, and Transverse Myelitis, as well as Primary Symptoms such as Fatigue, Spasticity, Tremors, Vocal Fold Paralysis, Optic Neuritis, Common Sleep Disorders, and Sexual Dysfunction

Along with Information on Treatment Options, Dietary Changes, Exercise Guidelines, Financial Planning, Legal Considerations, a Glossary of Terms Related to Multiple Sclerosis, and a Directory of Additional Resources

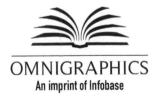

OMNIGRAPHICS
An imprint of Infobase

Bibliographic Note

Because this page cannot legibly accommodate all the copyright notices, the Bibliographic Note portion of the Preface constitutes an extension of the copyright notice.

* * *

OMNIGRAPHICS
An imprint of Infobase
8 The Green
Suite 19225
Dover, DE 19901
www.infobase.com
James Chambers, *Editorial Director*

* * *

Copyright © 2024 Infobase
ISBN 978-0-7808-2134-7
E-ISBN 978-0-7808-2135-4

Library of Congress Cataloging-in-Publication Data

Names: Chambers, James, editor.

Title: Multiple sclerosis sourcebook / James Chambers.

Description: Third edition. | Dover, DE: Omnigraphics, [2024] | Series: Health reference series | Includes index. | Summary: "Provides basic consumer health information about symptoms, diagnosis, treatment, and management of multiple sclerosis. Includes an index, glossary of related terms, and other resources"-- Provided by publisher.

Identifiers: LCCN 2024007836 (print) | LCCN 2024007837 (ebook) | ISBN 9780780821347 (library binding) | ISBN 9780780821354 (ebook)

Subjects: LCSH: Multiple sclerosis--Popular works.

Classification: LCC RC377 .M8638 2024 (print) | LCC RC377 (ebook) | DDC 616.8/34--dc23/eng/20240327

LC record available at https://lccn.loc.gov/2024007836

LC ebook record available at https://lccn.loc.gov/2024007837

Electronic or mechanical reproduction, including photography, recording, or any other information storage and retrieval system for the purpose of resale is strictly prohibited without permission in writing from the publisher.

The information in this publication was compiled from the sources cited and from other sources considered reliable. While every possible effort has been made to ensure reliability, the publisher will not assume liability for damages caused by inaccuracies in the data, and makes no warranty, express or implied, on the accuracy of the information contained herein.

This book is printed on acid-free paper meeting the ANSI Z39.48 Standard. The infinity symbol that appears above indicates that the paper in this book meets that standard.

Printed in the United States

Table of Contents

Preface ix

Part 1. Understanding Multiple Sclerosis
Chapter 1—Introduction to the Nervous System 3
Chapter 2—Overview of Multiple Sclerosis 17
Chapter 3—Causative Factors of Multiple Sclerosis 25
Chapter 4—Autoimmunity and Multiple Sclerosis 29
Chapter 5—Pregnancy and Multiple Sclerosis 33
Chapter 6—Variants of Multiple Sclerosis 37
            Section 6.1—Schilder Disease 39
            Section 6.2—Marburg Variant Multiple
                      Sclerosis 40
Chapter 7—Other Conditions Linked to Multiple Sclerosis 43
            Section 7.1—Chronic Inflammatory
                      Demyelinating Polyneuropathy 45
            Section 7.2—Neuromyelitis Optica 46
            Section 7.3—Transverse Myelitis 49
Chapter 8—NIH Study on Severe Multiple Sclerosis Risk 57
Chapter 9—Preventing Multiple Sclerosis in Children 61
Chapter 10—Managing Multiple Sclerosis Relapses 65

Part 2. Primary Symptoms of Multiple Sclerosis
Chapter 11—Fatigue 75
Chapter 12—Spasticity 79
Chapter 13—Tremors 83
Chapter 14—Pain 89
Chapter 15—Speech and Swallowing Problems 93

Chapter 16—Vocal Fold Paralysis 99
Chapter 17—Optic Neuritis 103
Chapter 18—Poor Balance 107
Chapter 19—Bladder Dysfunctions 111
Chapter 20—Cognitive Deficits 115
Chapter 21—Depression 121
Chapter 22—Common Sleep Disorders 125
Chapter 23—Sexual Dysfunction 129

Part 3. Diagnostic Tests, Treatments, and Therapies for Multiple Sclerosis

Chapter 24—Preparing for Annual Primary Care
    Evaluation 137
Chapter 25—Working with a Neurologist 141
Chapter 26—Diagnosing Multiple Sclerosis 147
    Section 26.1—Imaging Tests and Procedures
        for Multiple Sclerosis 149
    Section 26.2—Magnetic Resonance Imaging 151
    Section 26.3—Kurtzke Expanded Disability
        Status Scale 154
Chapter 27—Treatment Options for Multiple Sclerosis 159
Chapter 28—Plasmapheresis 171
Chapter 29—Vitamin D Therapy for Multiple Sclerosis 177
Chapter 30—Stem Cell Therapy for Multiple Sclerosis 181
Chapter 31—Halting Multiple Sclerosis Progression 185
Chapter 32—Complementary Approach for Multiple
    Sclerosis 189
Chapter 33—Rehabilitation Options for People with
    Multiple Sclerosis 193

Part 4. Living with Multiple Sclerosis

Chapter 34—Optimizing Life with Multiple Sclerosis 199
Chapter 35—Building Resilience 203
Chapter 36—Dietary Changes and Multiple Sclerosis 207

Chapter 37—Exercise Guidelines for Multiple Sclerosis 211
    Section 37.1—Creating Your Activity Plan
                  and Exercise Routine 213
    Section 37.2—Tips for Effective Exercise 218
Chapter 38—Link Between Bladder Dysfunction and Falls in
              Multiple Sclerosis 221
Chapter 39—Managing Bowel Issues 225
Chapter 40—Addressing Sexual Dysfunction 229
Chapter 41—Improving Sleep in Multiple Sclerosis 233
Chapter 42—Coping with Stress 237
Chapter 43—Fostering Effective Communication in
              Relationships 243
Chapter 44—Music Therapy for Multiple Sclerosis 247
Chapter 45—Temperature Sensitivity in Multiple Sclerosis 251
Chapter 46—Vaccinations for People with Multiple
              Sclerosis 259
Chapter 47—Dealing with Mobility Challenges 265
Chapter 48—Features of Home Accessibility 271
Chapter 49—Equipment for Self-Care and Independence 277
Chapter 50—Driving Considerations for People with
              Multiple Sclerosis 283
Chapter 51—Self-Advocacy and Effective Communication 287

Part 5. Multiple Sclerosis, Work, Financial, and Legal Issues
Chapter 52—Accommodating Employees with Multiple
              Sclerosis 293
Chapter 53—Disability Benefits for Multiple Sclerosis 299
Chapter 54—Building Support Networks with Multiple
              Sclerosis 311
Chapter 55—Long-Term Care Options and Multiple
              Sclerosis 315
Chapter 56—Guide to Disability Rights Laws 319
Chapter 57—Guardianship for People with Disability 329
Chapter 58—Advance Care Planning 335

Part 6. Additional Help and Information
Chapter 59—Glossary of Terms Related to Multiple Sclerosis 345
Chapter 60—Directory of Resources Providing Information
  about Multiple Sclerosis 351

Index 361

Preface

ABOUT THIS BOOK

Multiple sclerosis (MS) is the most prevalent acquired inflammatory demyelinating disorder affecting the central nervous system. Approximately 900,000 individuals in the United States and 2.3 million people worldwide are affected by the disease. It generally strikes people between the ages of 20 and 40 and frequently affects young adults and females. Symptoms of MS can vary significantly based on the location and severity of nerve damage but commonly include fatigue, muscle weakness, numbness or tingling, coordination and balance challenges, vision impairments, and cognitive changes. While a cure remains elusive, treatments exist to alleviate symptoms, slow disease progression, and enhance overall well-being.

Multiple Sclerosis Sourcebook, Third Edition provides comprehensive information about the causative factors, rare variants, primary symptoms, diagnostic tests, treatments, therapies, and management of MS. It delves into related conditions such as chronic inflammatory demyelinating polyneuropathy, neuromyelitis optica, and transverse myelitis. The book also covers various treatment options, including plasmapheresis, vitamin D therapy, and stem cell therapy, as well as complementary approaches and rehabilitation options. Additionally, it offers valuable insights into building resilience, dietary changes, exercise guidelines tailored for individuals with MS, and managing specific symptoms like bladder dysfunction, bowel issues, and sexual dysfunction. The book addresses the intersection of MS with work, financial, and legal issues, including information on disability benefits, long-term care options, and guardianship. It also emphasizes the importance of effective communication with health-care providers, strategies for coping with stress and depression, and maintaining overall well-being. The book concludes with a glossary of terms related to MS and a directory of organizations that provide additional information and support for patients and caregivers.

HOW TO USE THIS BOOK

This book is divided into parts and chapters. Parts focus on broad areas of interest. Chapters are devoted to single topics within a part.

Part 1: Understanding Multiple Sclerosis provides comprehensive information on the nervous system, factors causing multiple sclerosis (MS), the association between autoimmune diseases and MS, the prevalence of MS across different genders and ages, and variants of MS. It also covers other conditions connected to MS, such as chronic inflammatory demyelinating polyneuropathy, neuromyelitis optica, transverse myelitis, and trigeminal neuralgia.

Part 2: Primary Symptoms of Multiple Sclerosis explores various aspects of multiple sclerosis (MS), including fatigue, spasticity, communication challenges, cognitive impairments, vocal fold paralysis, balance issues affecting stability, and sexual dysfunction related to arousal and performance difficulties. It also addresses optic neuritis, pain, tremors, bladder dysfunction, and common sleep disorders.

Part 3: Diagnostic Tests, Treatments, and Therapies for Multiple Sclerosis covers the diagnosis of multiple sclerosis (MS) using magnetic resonance imaging (MRI) and the Kurtzke Expanded Disability Status Scale. It explores various treatment options aimed at halting MS progression, including disease-modifying therapies and emerging treatments. The part discusses plasmapheresis as a therapeutic approach and highlights the role of vitamin D in managing MS symptoms. It also addresses rehabilitation options, such as physical and occupational therapy, and includes insights into managing specific symptoms like bladder dysfunction, cognitive deficits, and spasticity.

Part 4: Living with Multiple Sclerosis provides comprehensive guidance on optimizing life with multiple sclerosis (MS). It includes information on dietary changes tailored for MS management, exercise guidelines to promote mobility and strength, the therapeutic benefits of music therapy, and the importance of vaccinations for individuals with MS. The part covers selecting and using equipment for daily self-care and enhancing independence. It also offers practical tips for managing specific symptoms like bladder and bowel dysfunction, sexual issues, and temperature sensitivity.

Part 5: Multiple Sclerosis, Work, Financial, and Legal Issues offers comprehensive support for individuals with multiple sclerosis (MS) across various life domains. It includes guidance on accommodating employees with MS in the workplace, financial planning considerations tailored to MS, health-care options for symptom management, understanding disability rights laws and accessing disability benefits, addressing guardianship needs for individuals with disabilities, and creating advance directives for medical decisions. The part also explores long-term care options, building support networks, and navigating legal aspects such as guardianship and advance care planning.

Part 6: Additional Help and Information includes a glossary of terms related to multiple sclerosis (MS) and a directory of resources providing further help and information.

BIBLIOGRAPHIC NOTE

This volume contains documents and excerpts from publications issued by the following U.S. government agencies: ADA.gov; Centers for Disease Control and Prevention (CDC); Centers for Medicare & Medicaid Services (CMS); *Eunice Kennedy Shriver* National Institute of Child Health and Human Development (NICHD); Genetic and Rare Diseases Information Center (GARD); MedlinePlus; National Center for Complementary and Integrative Health (NCCIH); National Council on Disability (NCD); National Institute of Arthritis and Musculoskeletal and Skin Diseases (NIAMS); National Institute of Mental Health (NIMH); National Institute of Neurological Disorders and Stroke (NINDS); National Institute on Aging (NIA); National Institute on Deafness and Other Communication Disorders (NIDCD); National Institutes of Health (NIH); *NIH News in Health*; Office of Disability Employment Policy (ODEP); Surveillance, Epidemiology, and End Results (SEER) Program; U.S. Department of Health and Human Services (HHS); U.S. Department of Veterans Affairs (VA); and U.S. Social Security Administration (SSA).

It also contains original material produced by Infobase.

ABOUT THE *HEALTH REFERENCE SERIES*

The *Health Reference Series* is designed to provide basic medical information for patients, families, caregivers, and the general public. Each volume provides comprehensive coverage on a particular topic. This is especially important for people who may be dealing with a newly diagnosed disease or a chronic disorder in themselves or in a family member. People looking for preventive guidance, information about disease warning signs, medical statistics, and risk factors for health problems will also find answers to their questions in the *Health Reference Series*. The *Series*, however, is not intended to serve as a tool for diagnosing illness, in prescribing treatments, or as a substitute for the physician-patient relationship. All people concerned about medical symptoms or the possibility of disease are encouraged to seek professional care from an appropriate health-care provider.

A NOTE ABOUT SPELLING AND STYLE

Health Reference Series editors use *Stedman's Medical Dictionary* as an authority for questions related to the spelling of medical terms and *The Chicago Manual of Style* for questions related to grammatical structures, punctuation, and other editorial concerns. Consistent adherence is not always possible, however, because the individual volumes within the *Series* include many documents from a wide variety of different producers, and the editor's primary goal is to present material from each source as accurately as is possible. This sometimes means that information in different chapters or sections may follow other guidelines and alternate spelling authorities. For example, occasionally a copyright holder may require that eponymous terms be shown in possessive forms (Crohn's disease vs. Crohn disease) or that British spelling norms be retained (leukaemia vs. leukemia).

HEALTH REFERENCE SERIES UPDATE POLICY

The inaugural book in the *Health Reference Series* was the first edition of *Cancer Sourcebook* published in 1989. Since then, the *Series* has been enthusiastically received by librarians and in the medical community. In order to maintain the standard of providing high-quality health information for the layperson, the editorial staff felt it was necessary to implement a policy of updating volumes when warranted.

Medical researchers have been making tremendous strides, and it is the purpose of the *Health Reference Series* to stay current with the most recent advances. Each decision to update a volume is made on an individual basis. Some of the considerations include how much new information is available and the feedback we receive from people who use the books. If there is a topic you would like to see added to the update list, or an area of medical concern you feel has not been adequately addressed, please write to: custserv@infobaselearning.com.

Part 1 | Understanding Multiple Sclerosis

Chapter 1 | Introduction to the Nervous System

The nervous system is the major controlling, regulatory, and communicating system in the body. It is the center of all mental activity including thought, learning, and memory. Together with the endocrine system, the nervous system is responsible for regulating and maintaining homeostasis. Through its receptors, the nervous system keeps us in touch with our environment, both external and internal.

Like other systems in the body, the nervous system is composed of organs, principally the brain, spinal cord, nerves, and ganglia. These, in turn, consist of various tissues, including nerve, blood, and connective tissue. Together these carry out the complex activities of the nervous system.[1]

The nervous system controls:
- brain growth and development
- sensations (such as touch or hearing)
- perception (the mental process of interpreting sensory information)
- thought and emotions
- learning and memory
- movement, balance, and coordination
- sleep
- healing and rehabilitation
- stress and the body's responses to stress
- aging

---

[1] Surveillance, Epidemiology, and End Results (SEER) Program, "Introduction to the Nervous System," National Cancer Institute (NCI), June 30, 2002. Available online. URL: https://training.seer.cancer.gov/anatomy/nervous. Accessed February 7, 2024.

- breathing and heartbeat
- body temperature
- hunger, thirst, and digestion
- puberty, reproductive health, and fertility[2]

The various activities of the nervous system can be grouped together as three general, overlapping functions:
- sensory
- integrative
- motor

Millions of sensory receptors detect changes, called "stimuli," which occur inside and outside the body. They monitor things such as temperature, light, and sound from the external environment. Inside the body, the internal environment, receptors detect variations in pressure, pH, carbon dioxide concentration, and the levels of various electrolytes. All of this gathered information is called "sensory input."

Sensory input is converted into electrical signals called "nerve impulses" that are transmitted to the brain. There the signals are brought together to create sensations, produce thoughts, or add to memory. Decisions are made each moment based on the sensory input. This is integration.

Based on the sensory input and integration, the nervous system responds by sending signals to muscles, causing them to contract, or to glands, causing them to produce secretions. Muscles and glands are called "effectors" because they cause an effect in response to directions from the nervous system. This is the motor output or motor function.

The nervous system also includes nonneuron cells, called "glia." Glia perform many important functions that keep the nervous system working properly. For example, glia:
- help support and hold neurons in place
- protect neurons

---

[2] "What Does the Nervous System Do?" *Eunice Kennedy Shriver* National Institute of Child Health and Human Development (NICHD), October 1, 2018. Available online. URL: www.nichd.nih.gov/health/topics/neuro/condition-info/functions. Accessed February 7, 2024.

Introduction to the Nervous System

- create insulation called "myelin," which helps move nerve impulses
- repair neurons and help restore neuron function
- trim out dead neurons
- regulate neurotransmitters

The brain is made up of many networks of communicating neurons and glia. These networks allow different parts of the brain to "talk" to each other and work together to control body functions, emotions, thinking, behavior, and other activities.[3]

NERVE TISSUE

Although the nervous system is very complex, there are only two main types of cells in nerve tissue. The actual nerve cell is the neuron. It is the "conducting" cell that transmits impulses and the structural unit of the nervous system. The other type of cell is the neuroglia, or glial, cell. The word "neuroglia" means "nerve glue." These cells are nonconductive and provide a support system for the neurons. They are a special type of "connective tissue" for the nervous system.

Neurons

Neurons, or nerve cells, carry out the functions of the nervous system by conducting nerve impulses. They are highly specialized and amitotic. This means that if a neuron is destroyed, it cannot be replaced because neurons do not go through mitosis. Figure 1.1 illustrates the structure of a typical neuron.

Each neuron has three basic parts, as described subsequently.

CELL BODY

In many ways, the cell body is similar to other types of cells. It has a nucleus with at least one nucleolus and contains many of the typical cytoplasmic organelles. It lacks centrioles, however. Because

---

[3] "What Are the Parts of the Nervous System?" *Eunice Kennedy Shriver* National Institute of Child Health and Human Development (NICHD), October 1, 2018. Available online. URL: www.nichd.nih.gov/health/topics/neuro/conditioninfo/parts. Accessed April 30, 2024.

centrioles function in cell division, the fact that neurons lack these organelles is consistent with the amitotic nature of the cell.

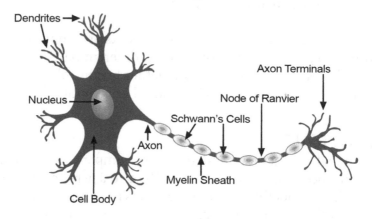

Figure 1.1. Structure of a Typical Neuron
National Cancer Institute (NCI)

DENDRITES

Dendrites and axons are cytoplasmic extensions, or processes, that project from the cell body. They are sometimes referred to as "fibers." Dendrites are usually, but not always, short and branching, which increases their surface area to receive signals from other neurons. The number of dendrites on a neuron varies. They are called "afferent processes" because they transmit impulses to the neuron cell body. There is only one axon that projects from each cell body. It is usually elongated and because it carries impulses away from the cell body, it is called an "efferent process."

AXON

An axon may have infrequent branches called "axon collaterals." Axons and axon collaterals terminate in many short branches or telodendria. The distal ends of the telodendria are slightly enlarged to form synaptic bulbs. Many axons are surrounded by a segmented, white, fatty substance called "myelin" or the "myelin sheath." Myelinated fibers make up the white matter in the central nervous system (CNS), while cell bodies and unmyelinated fibers make the gray matter. The unmyelinated regions between the myelin segments are called the "nodes of Ranvier."

In the peripheral nervous system (PNS), the myelin is produced by Schwann cells. The cytoplasm, nucleus, and outer cell membrane of the Schwann cell form a tight covering around the myelin and around the axon itself at the nodes of Ranvier. This covering is the neurilemma, which plays an important role in the regeneration of nerve fibers. In the CNS, oligodendrocytes produce myelin, but there is no neurilemma, which is why fibers within the CNS do not regenerate.

Functionally, neurons are classified as afferent, efferent, or interneurons (association neurons) according to the direction in which they transmit impulses relative to the CNS. Afferent, or sensory, neurons carry impulses from peripheral sense receptors to the CNS. They usually have long dendrites and relatively short axons. Efferent, or motor, neurons transmit impulses from the CNS to effector organs, such as muscles and glands. Efferent neurons usually have short dendrites and long axons. Interneurons, or association neurons, are located entirely within the CNS, in which they form the connecting link between the afferent and efferent neurons. They have short dendrites and may have either a short or long axon.

Neuroglia

Neuroglia cells do not conduct nerve impulses, but instead, they support, nourish, and protect the neurons. They are far more numerous than neurons and, unlike neurons, are capable of mitosis.

TUMORS

Schwannomas are benign tumors of the PNS that commonly occur in their sporadic, solitary form in otherwise normal individuals. Rarely, individuals develop multiple schwannomas arising from one or many elements of the PNS.

Commonly called a "Morton neuroma," this problem is a fairly common benign nerve growth and begins when the outer coating of a nerve in your foot thickens. This thickening is caused by irritation of branches of the medial and lateral plantar nerves that results when two bones repeatedly rub together.

ORGANIZATION OF THE NERVOUS SYSTEM

Although terminology seems to indicate otherwise, there is really only one nervous system in the body. Although each subdivision of the system is also called a "nervous system," all of these smaller systems belong to the single, highly integrated nervous system. Each subdivision has structural and functional characteristics that distinguish it from the others. The nervous system as a whole is divided into two subdivisions:

The Central Nervous System

The brain and spinal cord are the organs of the CNS. Because they are so vitally important, the brain and spinal cord, located in the dorsal body cavity, are encased in bone for protection. The brain is in the cranial vault, and the spinal cord is in the vertebral canal of the vertebral column. Although considered to be two separate organs, the brain and spinal cord are continuous at the foramen magnum.

The Peripheral Nervous System

The organs of the PNS are the nerves and ganglia. Nerves are bundles of nerve fibers, much like muscles are bundles of muscle fibers. Cranial nerves and spinal nerves extend from the CNS to peripheral organs, such as muscles and glands. Ganglia are collections, or small knots, of nerve cell bodies outside the CNS.

The PNS is further subdivided into an afferent (sensory) division and an efferent (motor) division. The afferent or sensory division transmits impulses from peripheral organs to the CNS. The efferent or motor division transmits impulses from the CNS out to the peripheral organs to cause an effect or action.

Finally, the efferent or motor division is again subdivided into the somatic nervous system and the autonomic nervous system. The somatic nervous system, also called the "somatomotor" or "somatic efferent nervous system," supplies motor impulses to the

Introduction to the Nervous System

skeletal muscles. Because these nerves permit conscious control of the skeletal muscles, it is sometimes called the "voluntary nervous system." The autonomic nervous system, also called the "visceral efferent nervous system," supplies motor impulses to cardiac muscle, smooth muscle, and glandular epithelium. It is further subdivided into sympathetic and parasympathetic divisions. Because the autonomic nervous system regulates involuntary or automatic functions, it is called the "involuntary nervous system."

THE CENTRAL NERVOUS SYSTEM

The CNS consists of the brain and spinal cord, which are located in the dorsal body cavity. The brain is surrounded by the cranium, and the spinal cord is protected by the vertebrae. The brain is continuous with the spinal cord at the foramen magnum. In addition to bone, the CNS is surrounded by connective tissue membranes, called "meninges," and by cerebrospinal fluid (CSF).

Figure 1.2 illustrates the intricate relationship between the brain and its surrounding structures, encompassing the skull, meninges, ventricles, and spinal cord.

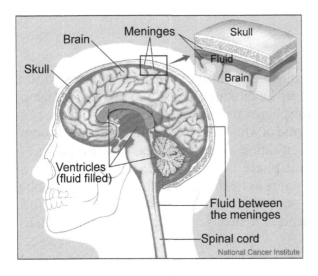

Figure 1.2. Brain and Nearby Structures
National Cancer Institute (NCI)

Meninges

There are three layers of meninges around the brain and spinal cord. The outer layer, the dura mater, is tough white fibrous connective tissue. The middle layer of meninges is arachnoid, which resembles a cobweb in appearance, and is a thin layer with numerous threadlike strands that attach it to the innermost layer. The space under the arachnoid, the subarachnoid space, is filled with CSF and contains blood vessels. The pia mater is the innermost layer of meninges. This thin, delicate membrane is tightly bound to the surface of the brain and spinal cord and cannot be dissected away without damaging the surface.

Meningiomas are tumors of the nerve tissue covering the brain and spinal cord. Although meningiomas are usually not likely to spread, physicians often treat them as though they were malignant to treat symptoms that may develop when a tumor applies pressure to the brain.

Brain

The brain is divided into cerebrum, diencephalon, brain stem, and cerebellum.

CEREBRUM

The largest and most obvious portion of the brain is the cerebrum, which is divided by a deep longitudinal fissure into two cerebral hemispheres. The two hemispheres are two separate entities but are connected by an arching band of white fibers, called the "corpus callosum" that provides a communication pathway between the two halves.

Each cerebral hemisphere is divided into five lobes, four of which have the same name as the bone over them: the frontal lobe, the parietal lobe, the occipital lobe, and the temporal lobe. A fifth lobe, the insula or Island of Reil, lies deep within the lateral sulcus.

DIENCEPHALON

The diencephalon is centrally located and is nearly surrounded by the cerebral hemispheres. It includes the thalamus, hypothalamus, and epithalamus. The thalamus, about 80 percent of the diencephalon, consists of two oval masses of gray matter that serve as relay stations for sensory impulses, except for the sense of smell, going to the cerebral cortex. The hypothalamus is a small region below the thalamus, which plays a key role in maintaining homeostasis because it regulates many visceral activities. The epithalamus is the most dorsal portion of the diencephalon. This small gland is involved with the onset of puberty and rhythmic cycles in the body. It is like a biological clock.

BRAIN STEM
The brain stem is the region between the diencephalon and the spinal cord. It consists of three parts: midbrain, pons, and medulla oblongata. The midbrain is the most superior portion of the brain stem. The pons is the bulging middle portion of the brain stem. This region primarily consists of nerve fibers that form conduction tracts between the higher brain centers and the spinal cord. The medulla oblongata, or simply medulla, extends inferiorly from the pons. It is continuous with the spinal cord at the foramen magnum. All the ascending (sensory) and descending (motor) nerve fibers connecting the brain and spinal cord pass through the medulla.

CEREBELLUM
The cerebellum, the second-largest portion of the brain, is located below the occipital lobes of the cerebrum. Three paired bundles of myelinated nerve fibers, called "cerebellar peduncles," form communication pathways between the cerebellum and other parts of the CNS.

VENTRICLES AND CEREBROSPINAL FLUID
A series of interconnected, fluid-filled cavities are found within the brain. These cavities are the ventricles of the brain, and the fluid is CSF.

SPINAL CORD
The spinal cord extends from the foramen magnum at the base of the skull to the level of the first lumbar vertebra. The cord is

continuous with the medulla oblongata at the foramen magnum. Like the brain, the spinal cord is surrounded by bone, meninges, and cerebrospinal fluid.

The spinal cord is divided into 31 segments with each segment giving rise to a pair of spinal nerves. At the distal end of the cord, many spinal nerves extend beyond the conus medullaris to form a collection that resembles a horse's tail. This is the cauda equina. In cross-section, the spinal cord appears oval.

The spinal cord has two main functions:
- **Serving as a conduction pathway for impulses going to and from the brain.** Sensory impulses travel to the brain on ascending tracts in the cord. Motor impulses travel on descending tracts.
- **Serving as a reflex center.** The reflex arc is the functional unit of the nervous system. Reflexes are responses to stimuli that do not require conscious thought and consequently, they occur more quickly than reactions that require thought processes. For example, with the withdrawal reflex, the reflex action withdraws the affected part before you are aware of the pain. Many reflexes are mediated in the spinal cord without going to the higher brain centers.

Brain Tumor

Glioma refers to tumors that arise from the support cells of the brain. These cells are called "glial cells." These tumors include the astrocytomas, ependymomas, and oligodendrogliomas. These tumors are the most common primary brain tumors.

THE PERIPHERAL NERVOUS SYSTEM

The PNS consists of the nerves that branch out from the brain and spinal cord. These nerves form the communication network between the CNS and the body parts. The PNS is further subdivided into the somatic nervous system and the autonomic nervous system. The somatic nervous system consists of nerves that go to the skin and muscles and are involved in conscious activities. The autonomic nervous system consists of nerves that connect the CNS to the visceral organs, such as the heart, stomach, and intestines. It mediates unconscious activities.

Structure of a Nerve

A nerve contains bundles of nerve fibers, either axons or dendrites, surrounded by connective tissue. Sensory nerves contain only afferent fibers, long dendrites of sensory neurons. Motor nerves have only efferent fibers, long axons of motor neurons. Mixed nerves contain both types of fibers.

A connective tissue sheath called the "epineurium" surrounds each nerve. Each bundle of nerve fibers is called a "fasciculus" and is surrounded by a layer of connective tissue called the "perineurium." Within the fasciculus, each individual nerve fiber, with its myelin and neurilemma, is surrounded by connective tissue called the "endoneurium." A nerve may also have blood vessels enclosed in its connective tissue wrappings.

Cranial Nerves

Twelve pairs of cranial nerves emerge from the inferior surface of the brain. All of these nerves, except the vagus nerve, pass through the foramina of the skull to innervate structures in the head, neck, and facial region.

The cranial nerves are designated both by name and by Roman numerals, according to the order in which they appear on the inferior surface of the brain. Most of the nerves have both sensory and motor components. Three of the nerves are associated with the special senses of smell, vision, hearing, and equilibrium and have only sensory fibers. Five other nerves are primarily motor in function but do have some sensory fibers for proprioception. The remaining four nerves consist of significant amounts of both sensory and motor fibers.

Acoustic neuromas are benign fibrous growths that arise from the balance nerve, also called the "eighth cranial nerve" or "vestibulocochlear nerve." These tumors are nonmalignant, they do not spread or metastasize to other parts of the body. The location of these tumors is deep inside the skull, adjacent to vital brain centers in the brain stem. As the tumors enlarge, they involve surrounding structures that have to do with vital functions. In the majority of cases, these tumors grow slowly over a period of years. In other cases, the growth rate is more rapid and patients develop symptoms at a faster pace. Usually, the symptoms are mild, and many patients are not diagnosed until some time after their tumor has developed. Many patients also exhibit no tumor growth over a number of years when followed by yearly magnetic resonance imaging (MRI) scans.

Spinal Nerves

Thirty-one pairs of spinal nerves emerge laterally from the spinal cord. Each pair of nerves corresponds to a segment of the cord, and they are named accordingly. This means there are 8 cervical nerves, 12 thoracic nerves, 5 lumbar nerves, 5 sacral nerves, and 1 coccygeal nerve.

Each spinal nerve is connected to the spinal cord by a dorsal root and a ventral root. The cell bodies of the sensory neurons are in the dorsal root ganglion, but the motor neuron cell bodies are in the gray matter. The two roots join to form the spinal nerve just before the nerve leaves the vertebral column. Because all spinal nerves have both sensory and motor components, they are all mixed nerves.

Autonomic Nervous System

The autonomic nervous system is a visceral efferent system, which means it sends motor impulses to the visceral organs. It functions automatically and continuously, without conscious effort, to innervate smooth muscle, cardiac muscle, and glands. It is concerned with heart rate, breathing rate, blood pressure, body temperature, and other visceral activities that work together to maintain homeostasis.

Introduction to the Nervous System

The autonomic nervous system has two parts, the sympathetic division and the parasympathetic division. Many visceral organs are supplied with fibers from both divisions. In this case, one stimulates and the other inhibits. This antagonistic functional relationship serves as a balance to help maintain homeostasis.[4]

Studying and understanding the nervous system is important because it affects so many areas of human health and well-being.[5]

---

[4] See footnote [1].
[5] See footnote [2].

Chapter 2 | Overview of Multiple Sclerosis

Multiple sclerosis (MS) is a condition characterized by areas of damage (lesions) on the brain and spinal cord. These lesions are associated with destruction of the covering that protects nerves and promotes the efficient transmission of nerve impulses (the myelin sheath) and damage to nerve cells (see Figure 2.1). MS is considered an autoimmune disorder; autoimmune disorders occur when the immune system malfunctions and attacks the body's own tissues and organs, in this case tissues of the nervous system. MS usually begins in early adulthood, between ages 20 and 40.[1]

WHAT ARE THE SIGNS AND SYMPTOMS OF MULTIPLE SCLEROSIS?
The natural course of MS is different for each person, which makes it difficult to predict. The onset and duration of MS symptoms usually depends on the specific type but may begin over a few days and go away quickly or develop more slowly and gradually over many years.

There are four main types of MS, named according to the progression of symptoms over time:
- **Relapsing-remitting MS.** Symptoms in this type come in attacks and, in-between attacks, people recover or return to their usual level of ability. The occurrence of symptoms in this form of MS is called an "attack" or, in medical terms, a "relapse" or "exacerbation." The

---

[1] MedlinePlus, "Multiple Sclerosis," National Institutes of Health (NIH), October 1, 2015. Available online. URL: https://medlineplus.gov/genetics/condition/multiple-sclerosis. Accessed February 16, 2024.

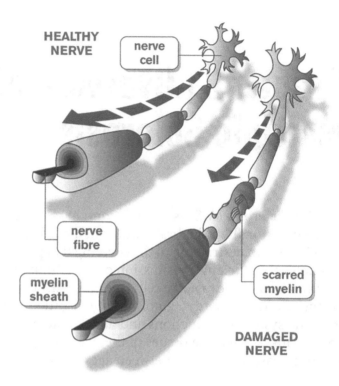

Figure 2.1. Healthy Nerve versus MS Nerve

U.S. Department of Veterans Affairs (VA)

periods of disease inactivity or quiescence between MS attacks is referred to as "remission." Weeks, months, or even years may pass before another attack occurs, followed again by a period of inactivity. Most people with MS (approximately 80%) are initially diagnosed with this form of the disease.

- **Secondary-progressive MS.** People with this form of MS usually have had a previous history of MS attacks but then start to develop gradual and steady symptoms and deterioration in their function over time. Most individuals with severe relapsing-remitting MS may go on to develop secondary-progressive MS if they are untreated.

Overview of Multiple Sclerosis

- **Primary-progressive MS.** This type of MS is less common and is characterized by progressively worsening symptoms from the beginning with no noticeable relapses or exacerbations of the disease, although there may be temporary or minor relief from symptoms.
- **Progressive-relapsing MS.** This rarest form of MS is characterized by a steady worsening of symptoms from the beginning, with acute relapses that can occur over time during the disease course.

There are some rare and unusual variants of MS. One of these is Marburg variant MS (also called "malignant MS"), which causes swift and relentless symptoms and decline in function, which can result in significant disability or even death shortly after disease onset. Balo's concentric sclerosis, which causes concentric rings of myelin destruction that can be seen on magnetic resonance imaging (MRI), is another variant type of MS that can progress rapidly.

Early MS symptoms often include the following:
- vision problems such as blurred or double vision, or optic neuritis, which causes pain with eye movement and a rapid loss of vision
- muscle weakness, often in the hands and legs, and muscle stiffness accompanied by painful muscle spasms
- tingling, numbness, or pain in the arms, legs, trunk, or face
- clumsiness, particularly difficulty staying balanced when walking
- bladder control problems
- intermittent or more constant dizziness

MS may also cause later symptoms such as:
- mental or physical fatigue which accompanies the early symptoms during an attack
- mood changes such as depression or difficulty with emotional expression or control
- cognitive dysfunction—problems concentrating, multitasking, thinking, learning, or difficulties with memory or judgment

Muscle weakness, stiffness, and spasms may be severe enough to affect walking or standing. In some cases, MS leads to partial or complete paralysis and the use of a wheelchair is not uncommon, particularly in individuals who are untreated or have advanced disease. Many people with MS find that weakness and fatigue are worse when they have a fever or when they are exposed to heat. MS exacerbations may occur following common infections.

Pain is rarely the first sign of MS, but pain often occurs with optic neuritis and trigeminal neuralgia, a disorder that affects one of the nerves that provides sensation to different parts of the face. Painful limb spasms and sharp pain shooting down the legs or around the abdomen can also be symptoms of MS.

Many individuals with MS may experience difficulties with coordination and balance. Some may have a continuous trembling of the head, limbs, and body, especially during movement.

MULTIPLE SCLEROSIS EXACERBATION

An exacerbation—which is also called a "relapse," "flare-up," or "attack"—is a sudden worsening of MS symptoms or the appearance of new symptoms that lasts for at least 24 hours. MS relapses are thought to be associated with the development of new areas of damage in the brain. Exacerbations are characteristic of relapsing-remitting MS.

An exacerbation may be mild or severe enough to significantly interfere with life's daily activities. Most exacerbations last from several days to several weeks, although some have lasted for as long as a few months. When the symptoms of the attack subside, an individual with MS is said to be in remission, characterized by disease quiescence.[2]

Corticosteroids

The standard treatment for MS relapses associated with significant disability is high-dose corticosteroids for three to five days. This

---

[2] "Multiple Sclerosis: Hope through Research," National Institute of Neurological Disorders and Stroke (NINDS), August 2020. Available online. URL: https://catalog.ninds.nih.gov/sites/default/files/publications/multiple-sclerosis-hope-through-research_0.pdf. Accessed February 16, 2024.

is usually 1,000 mg of intravenous methylprednisolone (IVMP) in 100 cc of normal saline over one hour daily for three to five days. Intravenous dexamethasone at 140 to 200 mg/day for three to five days is occasionally used in place of IVMP in cases of allergy or intolerance of methylprednisolone or oral prednisone at 1,250 mg/day for three to five days if intravenous treatment is not practical. The high-dose corticosteroids may be followed by a short taper of oral prednisone, but this oral steroid taper has unclear benefits.

Plasma Exchange

For severe MS relapses that do not respond to high-dose corticosteroids, plasma exchange may be considered. The side effects of plasma exchange must be balanced against the severity of symptoms. This treatment usually requires hospitalization. A course of treatment consists of plasma exchange every other day for five treatments. Others use daily plasma exchange for five treatments.

Rehabilitation

Relapse management may also include rehabilitation such as physical, occupational, or speech therapy to help with symptom management and potentially lessen the overall effects of the acute neurological event and any problems remaining after the relapse.[3]

FREQUENCY

An estimated 1.1–2.5 million people worldwide have MS. Although the reason is unclear, this condition is more common in regions that are farther away from the equator. In Canada, parts of the Northern United States, Western and Northern Europe, Russia, and Southeastern Australia, the condition affects approximately 1 in 2,000–2,400 people. It is less common closer to the equator, such as in Asia, sub-Saharan Africa, and parts of South America, where about 1 in 20,000 people are affected. For unknown reasons,

---

[3] "Treatments for Multiple Sclerosis Relapses," U.S. Department of Veterans Affairs (VA), February 13, 2024. Available online. URL: www.va.gov/MS/TREATING_MS/Treatments_for_Multiple_Sclerosis_Relapses.asp. Accessed April 25, 2024.

most forms of MS affect women twice as often as men; however, women and men are equally affected by primary-progressive MS.

CAUSES

Although the cause of MS is unknown, variations in dozens of genes are thought to be involved in MS risk. Changes in the human leukocyte antigen class II histocompatibility, D related beta chain (*HLA-DRB1*) gene are the strongest genetic risk factors for developing MS. Other factors associated with an increased risk of developing MS include changes in the interleukin 7 receptor (*IL7R*) gene and environmental factors, such as exposure to the Epstein-Barr virus (EBV), low levels of vitamin D, and smoking.

The *HLA-DRB1* gene belongs to a family of genes called the "human leukocyte antigen" (HLA) complex. The HLA complex helps the immune system distinguish the body's own proteins from proteins made by foreign invaders (such as viruses and bacteria). Each *HLA* gene has many different normal variations, allowing each person's immune system to react to a wide range of foreign proteins. Variations in several *HLA* genes have been associated with increased MS risk, but one particular variant of the *HLA-DRB1* gene, called "*HLA-DRB1*15:01*," is the most strongly linked genetic factor.

The *IL7R* gene provides instructions for making one piece of two different receptor proteins: the interleukin 7 (IL-7) receptor and the thymic stromal lymphopoietin (TSLP) receptor. Both receptors are embedded in the cell membrane of immune cells. These receptors stimulate signaling pathways that induce the growth and division (proliferation) and survival of immune cells. The genetic variation involved in MS leads to the production of an IL-7 receptor that is not embedded in the cell membrane but is instead found inside the cell. It is unknown if this variation affects the TSLP receptor.

Because the *HLA-DRB1* and *IL-7R* genes are involved in the immune system, changes in either might be related to the autoimmune response that damages the myelin sheath and nerve cells and leads to the signs and symptoms of MS. However, it is unclear exactly what role variations in either gene plays in development of the condition.

INHERITANCE

The inheritance pattern of MS is unknown, although the condition does appear to be passed down through generations in families. The risk of developing MS is higher for siblings or children of a person with the condition than for the general population.[4]

Most people with MS, however, will have short periods of symptoms followed by long stretches of relative quiescence (inactivity or dormancy), with partial or full recovery. Women are affected more frequently with MS compared to men. The disease is rarely fatal, and most people with MS have a normal life expectancy. New treatments can reduce long-term disability for many people with MS. Currently, there are still no cures and no clear ways to prevent the disease from developing.[5]

---

[4] See footnote [1].
[5] See footnote [2].

Chapter 3 | Causative Factors of Multiple Sclerosis

Researchers are looking at several possible explanations for why the immune system attacks the central nervous system (CNS) myelin, including:
- fighting an infectious agent (e.g., a virus) that has components that mimic components of the brain (called "molecular mimicry")
- destroying brain cells because they are unhealthy
- mistakenly identifying normal brain cells as foreign

There is also something known as the "blood-brain barrier" (BBB), which separates the brain and spinal cord from the immune system. If there is a break in this barrier, it exposes the brain to the immune system. When this happens, the immune system may misinterpret structures in the brain, such as myelin, as "foreign." Research shows that genetic vulnerabilities combined with environmental factors may cause multiple sclerosis (MS).

GENETIC SUSCEPTIBILITY

MS itself is not inherited, but susceptibility to MS may be inherited. Studies show that some individuals with MS have one or more family member or relative who also have MS.

Current research suggests that dozens of genes and possibly hundreds of variations in the genetic code (called "gene variants") combine to create vulnerability to MS. Some of these genes have been identified, and most are associated with functions of the immune system. Many of the known genes are similar to those that have been identified in people with other autoimmune diseases such as type 1 diabetes, rheumatoid arthritis (RA), or lupus.

INFECTIOUS FACTORS AND VIRUSES

Several viruses have been found in people with MS, but the virus most consistently linked to the development of MS is the Epstein-Barr virus (EBV), which causes infectious mononucleosis. Only about 5 percent of the population has not been infected by EBV. These individuals are at a lower risk for developing MS than those who have been infected. People who were infected with EBV in adolescence or adulthood and who therefore develop an exaggerated immune response to EBV are at a significantly higher risk for developing MS than those who were infected in early childhood. This suggests that it may be the type of immune response to EBV that may lead to MS, rather than EBV infection itself. However, there is still no proof that EBV causes MS, and the mechanisms that underlie this process are poorly understood.

ENVIRONMENTAL FACTORS

Several studies indicate that people who spend more time in the sun and those with relatively higher levels of vitamin D are less likely to develop MS or have a less severe course of disease and fewer relapses. Bright sunlight helps human skin produce vitamin D. Researchers believe that vitamin D may help regulate the immune system in ways that reduce the risk of MS or autoimmunity in general. People from regions near the equator, where there is a great deal of bright sunlight, generally have a much lower risk of MS than people from temperate areas such as the United States and Canada.

Causative Factors of Multiple Sclerosis

Studies have found that people who smoke are more likely to develop MS and have a more aggressive disease course. People who smoke tend to have more brain lesions and brain shrinkage than nonsmokers. The reasons for this are currently unclear.[1]

---

[1] "Multiple Sclerosis: Hope through Research," National Institute of Neurological Disorders and Stroke (NINDS), August 15, 2020. Available online. URL: https://catalog.ninds.nih.gov/sites/default/files/publications/multiple-sclerosis-hope-through-research_0.pdf. Accessed February 16, 2024.

Chapter 4 | Autoimmunity and Multiple Sclerosis

Your immune system is the network of cells and tissues in your body that works together to defend you from viruses, bacteria, and infection. It tries to identify and destroy the invaders that might hurt you.

In autoimmune diseases, proteins known as "autoantibodies" target the body's own healthy tissues by mistake, signaling the body to attack them.[1]

Multiple sclerosis (MS) is a disease in which the body's immune system inappropriately attacks the brain and spinal cord. Specifically, the immune system targets the fatty insulating material around nerves called "myelin." When myelin is damaged, the messages that nerve cells send and receive can be interrupted.[2]

MYELIN AND THE IMMUNE SYSTEM

Multiple sclerosis attacks axons in the central nervous system (CNS) protected by myelin, which are commonly called "white matter." MS also damages the nerve cell bodies, which are found in the brain's gray matter, as well as the axons themselves in the brain, spinal cord, and optic nerves that transmit visual information from the eye to the brain. As the disease progresses, the outermost layer of the brain, called the "cerebral cortex," shrinks (what is known

---

[1] "Autoimmune Diseases," National Institute of Arthritis and Musculoskeletal and Skin Diseases (NIAMS), March 2023. Available online. URL: www.niams.nih.gov/health-topics/autoimmune-diseases. Accessed February 16, 2024.
[2] *NIH News in Health,* "The Mystery of Multiple Sclerosis," National Institutes of Health (NIH), March 2011. Available online. URL: https://newsinhealth.nih.gov/2011/03/mystery-multiple-sclerosis. Accessed February 16, 2024.

Multiple Sclerosis Sourcebook, Third Edition

as "cortical atrophy"). Figure 4.1 shows normal, healthy axon and damaged proteins in the myelin sheath.

The term multiple sclerosis refers to the distinctive areas of scar tissue (sclerosis—also called "plaques" or "lesions") that result from the attack on myelin by the immune system. These plaques are visible using magnetic resonance imaging (MRI) in the white and/or gray matter of people who have MS. Plaques can be as small as a pinhead or as large as a golf ball.

During an MS exacerbation, most of the myelin, and to a lesser extent the axons within the affected area, is damaged or destroyed by different types of immune cells (also known as "inflammation"). The symptoms of MS depend on the severity of the inflammatory

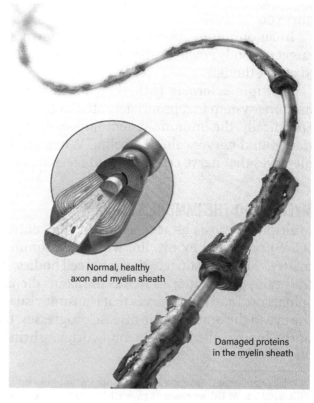

Normal, healthy axon and myelin sheath

Damaged proteins in the myelin sheath

Figure 4.1. Myelin Sheath
National Institute of Neurological Disorders and Stroke (NINDS)

reaction as well as the location and extent of the plaques, which primarily appear in the brain stem, cerebellum (involved with balance and coordination of movement, among other functions), spinal cord, optic nerves, and the white matter around the brain ventricles (fluid-filled spaces).[3]

THE MYSTERY OF MULTIPLE SCLEROSIS

Researchers estimate that 250,000 to 350,000 people in the United States have been diagnosed with MS. Scientists do not understand yet what triggers the immune system to attack myelin in these people. But researchers do know that Whites are more than twice as likely as others to develop MS, and women almost twice as likely as men.[4]

MS is a chronic disease that affects people differently. A small number of those with MS will have a mild course with little to no disability, whereas others will have a steadily worsening disease that leads to increased disability over time.[5]

---

[3] "Multiple Sclerosis: Hope through Research," National Institute of Neurological Disorders and Stroke (NINDS), August 15, 2020. Available online. URL: https://catalog.ninds.nih.gov/sites/default/files/publications/multiple-sclerosis-hope-through-research_0.pdf. Accessed February 16, 2024.
[4] See footnote [2].
[5] See footnote [3].

Chapter 5 | Pregnancy and Multiple Sclerosis

Multiple sclerosis (MS) affects women nearly three times as often as men, and often presents during childbearing years, making pregnancy issues very important for people living with MS. Questions around pregnancy and MS are a common part of patient-physician conversations.

EFFECT OF PREGNANCY ON MULTIPLE SCLEROSIS

Since MS is usually diagnosed in individuals between the ages of 20 and 40, the effect of pregnancy on MS is an important concern. Fortunately, MS is typically least likely to relapse during pregnancy. Several reasons probably account for this, including immunological changes thought to protect the developing fetus. Reduced disease activity during pregnancy also occurs with some other autoimmune diseases, such as psoriasis and rheumatoid arthritis (RA). The hormonal changes accompanying pregnancy, such as increasing levels of estradiol and estriol, peak in the third trimester, and these peaks correlate with decreased risk of MS activity during this time by as much as 70 percent. So although these changes likely are meant to protect the developing baby, these changes are also protective for the mother.

Another consideration for women with MS planning pregnancy is concern about fatigue, a very common symptom for any expectant mother. Fatigue is also one of the most common symptoms of MS. In nonpregnant women with MS, numerous medications can be used to manage fatigue, but these are not considered safe during pregnancy. To combat fatigue, it is important to allow for adequate rest and pay close attention to overall health during pregnancy. Watching for urinary tract infections as well as preventing pregnancy-associated anemia by taking prenatal vitamins with iron supplementation are some practical ways to reduce pregnancy-associated fatigue, which may compound MS fatigue.

Over the longer term, people with MS may wonder about the effect of the number of pregnancies on their MS progression. Studies thus far do not show worsening of an individual's overall MS course based on the number of pregnancies. Additionally, one study showed that having one or more pregnancies was associated with a lower risk of developing MS than having no pregnancies at all. While this is only one study, this is encouraging for women with MS who are considering having a child, but of course pregnancy is not a sustainable treatment for MS and does not substitute for disease modifying treatments (DMTs).

For those who do experience MS relapse during pregnancy, intravenous steroids (methylprednisolone) or intravenous immunoglobulin (IVIG) can be used. Coordination of care between the treating neurologist and obstetrics and gynecology (OB/GYN) is important should this occur.

EFFECT OF MULTIPLE SCLEROSIS ON PREGNANCY

People with MS do not have an increase in pregnancy complications due to MS, such as premature delivery. In general, there is no evidence of an association between maternal MS and adverse effects on fetal development.

Ten to fifteen percent of people in the United States have impaired fertility and the number is similar for people with MS. Some people with more progressive MS may experience sexual dysfunction, which could lead to impaired fertility, and this may require more specific management with counseling and possibly physical therapy and/or medications. People with MS who do experience infertility may need to use assisted reproductive technology (ART), and these approaches can be associated with a slight, temporary increased risk of MS relapse.

Since unplanned pregnancies do occur, it is important for people with MS to know that there is no evidence for any negative effect from use of contraceptives on MS disease course. For many, use of long-acting reversible contraceptives (LARCs), such as intrauterine devices (IUDs), are particularly helpful, since the risks of noncompliance are reduced, and this results in fewer unintended pregnancies. In general, any form of contraception is safe for people with MS. This is important to discuss with either a primary care provider or obstetrician and gynecologist.

BREASTFEEDING AND POSTPARTUM CONSIDERATIONS

Typically, the benefits of pregnancy with regard to the lower MS relapse rate rapidly diminishes postpartum, with risk of MS relapse peaking at around three to six months after delivery. There is no sufficient consistent evidence currently that supports not resuming DMT in that time frame in women with MS, particularly those with very active disease. Since DMTs vary in safety during lactation, as well as how quickly a therapeutic benefit occurs after resuming these medications, people with MS and physicians should be prepared early by discussing before delivery how and when to restart medications.

Often, a magnetic resonance imaging (MRI) will help guide these discussions because MRI can provide information about how active MS disease is postpartum. Gadolinium use during pregnancy is controversial but if given during lactation very little would be expected to be absorbed by the infant. There is no need to interrupt breastfeeding after gadolinium administration. Timing of postpartum MRI should be based on clinical status of the mother, as well as breastfeeding and family planning goals but would be urgently indicated if an acute relapse occurs.

It is recommended that people with MS must have adequate serum vitamin D levels, particularly during pregnancy, as this is associated with lower risk of MS relapses in mothers with MS and lower risk of developing MS in their offspring.[1]

---

[1] "Pregnancy in Multiple Sclerosis," U.S. Department of Veterans Affairs (VA), February 13, 2024. Available online. URL: www.va.gov/MS/Veterans/symptoms_of_MS/Pregnancy_in_Multiple_Sclerosis.asp. Accessed February 19, 2024.

Chapter 6 | Variants of Multiple Sclerosis

Chapter Contents
Section 6.1—Schilder Disease 39
Section 6.2—Marburg Variant Multiple Sclerosis 40

Section 6.1 | Schilder Disease

WHAT IS SCHILDER DISEASE?
Schilder disease, also known as "myelinoclastic diffuse sclerosis," is an extremely rare disease that involves the breakdown of the protective coating (called "myelin") over nerves in the brain and spinal cord.

WHO IS AFFECTED BY SCHILDER DISEASE?
The disease typically begins in childhood or adolescence and slowly gets worse. Lesions form in each half of the brain.

ARE SCHILDER DISEASE AND ADDISON-SCHILDER DISEASE THE SAME?
Schilder disease is not the same as Addison-Schilder disease, a form of adrenoleukodystrophy (a genetic disorder that involves damage to myelin).

WHAT CAUSES SCHILDER DISEASE?
The cause of Schilder disease is unknown, but scientists think it may be a type of multiple sclerosis (MS).

WHAT ARE THE SYMPTOMS OF SCHILDER DISEASE?
Symptoms of Schilder disease may include:
- weakness on one side of the body
- difficulty with speech (dysarthria)
- stiff muscles
- problems with balance
- headache
- seizures
- personality changes
- problems with hearing or vision
- loss of bowel or bladder control
- dementia

WHAT ARE THE TREATMENTS FOR SCHILDER DISEASE?
Treatment generally follows the established standards in MS and may include corticosteroids, interferon beta or immunosuppressive therapy, and symptomatic treatment.

CAN SCHILDER DISEASE BE CURED?
Currently, the disease has no cure.[1]

Section 6.2 | Marburg Variant Multiple Sclerosis

WHAT IS MARBURG VARIANT MULTIPLE SCLEROSIS?
Marburg variant multiple sclerosis (MS), also known as "malignant MS," is an aggressive and rare form of MS. It is characterized by rapidly progressive inflammation and destruction of myelin (protective covering surrounding the nerves) and increased formation of lesions and plaque in the brain and spine. The loss of myelin affects the brain's ability to transmit electrochemical impulses between the nerve cells of the brain and the spinal cord, resulting in deterioration or loss of neurological functioning.

As the disease progresses, lesions develop in the areas of the brain responsible for information processing, resulting in cognitive impairments such as difficulties with concentration, attention, memory, language, and judgment. People with malignant MS can have damage to regions of the brain responsible for behavior and emotions resulting in psychotic disorders such as manic depression and paranoia.

SYMPTOMS OF MARBURG VARIANT MULTIPLE SCLEROSIS
Physical symptoms may include:
- weakness in the extremities
- difficulties with coordination and balance

---

[1] "Schilder's Disease," National Institute of Neurological Disorders and Stroke (NINDS), November 28, 2023. Available online. URL: www.ninds.nih.gov/health-information/disorders/schilders-disease. Accessed February 14, 2024.

Variants of Multiple Sclerosis

- spasticity
- paresthesias (abnormal sensory feelings of numbness and prickling sensations)
- speech impediments
- tremors
- dizziness
- hearing loss
- vision impairments
- bowel and bladder difficulties

DIAGNOSIS OF MARBURG VARIANT MULTIPLE SCLEROSIS

There is no single test to detect malignant MS. It may be difficult to distinguish between a diagnosis of malignant MS and acute disseminated encephalomyelitis (ADEM) because of the timing of the occurrence of plaques in the brain tissue. A neurological exam is performed to assess symptoms and to rule out other possible disorders. Analysis of the cerebrospinal fluid (CSF) is also helpful for the diagnosis of malignant MS. Neuroimaging technologies, such as magnetic resonance imaging (MRI), diffusion-tensor magnetic resonance imaging (DT-MRI), and computerized brain tomography are used to detect central nervous system (CNS) lesions, myelin loss, white matter abnormalities, and other physical changes in the brain.

TREATMENT FOR MARBURG VARIANT MULTIPLE SCLEROSIS

There is currently no cure for malignant MS. Treatment generally consists of immunomodulatory therapy and the management of symptoms. Physical and occupational therapies can help the person perform daily activities such as handwriting, buttoning, and using eating utensils. Ambulatory aids such as canes, walkers, and wheelchairs are prescribed for gait and ataxia.

PROGNOSIS OF MARBURG VARIANT MULTIPLE SCLEROSIS

People with malignant MS experience a rapid decline in functioning. They require assistance with ambulation within five years from symptom onset due to the loss of the ability of the nerve cell (neurons) to transmit impulses to muscles that control motor functioning. Assistance with activities of daily living (ADLs) is required.[2]

---

[2] "Malignant Multiple Sclerosis," U.S. Social Security Administration (SSA), September 16, 2020. Available online. URL: https://secure.ssa.gov/poms.nsf/lnx/0423022620. Accessed February 14, 2024.

Chapter 7 | Other Conditions Linked to Multiple Sclerosis

Chapter Contents
Section 7.1—Chronic Inflammatory Demyelinating
 Polyneuropathy..45
Section 7.2—Neuromyelitis Optica...46
Section 7.3—Transverse Myelitis..49

Section 7.1 | Chronic Inflammatory Demyelinating Polyneuropathy

WHAT IS CHRONIC INFLAMMATORY DEMYELINATING POLYNEUROPATHY?
Chronic inflammatory demyelinating polyneuropathy (CIDP) is a neurological disorder that involves progressive weakness and reduced senses in the arms and legs.

SYMPTOMS OF CHRONIC INFLAMMATORY DEMYELINATING POLYNEUROPATHY
The symptoms of CIDP are:
- tingling or no feeling in fingers and toes
- weakness of arms and legs
- loss of deep tendon (muscle stretch) reflexes
- fatigue or feeling tired
- unusual feelings in the body

WHAT CAUSES CHRONIC INFLAMMATORY DEMYELINATING POLYNEUROPATHY
Chronic inflammatory demyelinating polyneuropathy is caused by damage to the fat-based protective covering on nerves called the "myelin sheath."

WHO IS AFFECTED BY CHRONIC INFLAMMATORY DEMYELINATING POLYNEUROPATHY?
Chronic inflammatory demyelinating polyneuropathy can happen at any age and in both genders but is more common in young adult men.

IS THERE A RELATIONSHIP BETWEEN CHRONIC INFLAMMATORY DEMYELINATING POLYNEUROPATHY AND GUILLAIN-BARRÉ SYNDROME?
Chronic inflammatory demyelinating polyneuropathy is closely related to Guillain-Barré syndrome (in which the immune system

mistakenly attacks the body) and is considered the long-term part of that disease.

TREATMENT FOR CHRONIC INFLAMMATORY DEMYELINATING POLYNEUROPATHY

Treatment for CIDP includes the use of steroid medicine and other treatments that focus on the immune system, along with physical therapy.[1]

Section 7.2 | Neuromyelitis Optica

WHAT IS NEUROMYELITIS OPTICA?

Neuromyelitis optica (NMO) is an autoimmune disorder that affects the nerves of the eyes and the central nervous system (CNS), which includes the brain and spinal cord. NMO is characterized by optic neuritis, which is inflammation of the nerve that carries information from the eye to the brain (optic nerve). Optic neuritis causes eye pain and vision loss, which can occur in one or both eyes.

SIGNS AND SYMPTOMS OF NEUROMYELITIS OPTICA

Approximately one-quarter of individuals with NMO have signs or symptoms of another autoimmune disorder, such as myasthenia gravis (MG), systemic lupus erythematosus (SLE), or Sjögren syndrome (SS). Some scientists believe that a condition described in Japanese patients as "optic-spinal multiple sclerosis" (or "opticospinal multiple sclerosis") that affects the nerves of the eyes and CNS is the same as NMO.

---

[1] "Chronic Inflammatory Demyelinating Polyneuropathy (CIDP)," National Institute of Neurological Disorders and Stroke (NINDS), November 28, 2023. Available online. URL: www.ninds.nih.gov/health-information/disorders/chronic-inflammatory-demyelinating-polyneuropathy-cidp. Accessed February 16, 2024.

CAUSES OF NEUROMYELITIS OPTICA

No genes associated with NMO have been identified. However, a small percentage of people with this condition have a family member who is also affected, which indicates that there may be one or more genetic changes that increase susceptibility. It is thought that the inheritance of this condition is complex and that many environmental and genetic factors are involved in the development of the condition.

The aquaporin-4 (AQP4) protein, a normal protein in the body, plays a role in NMO. The AQP4 is found in several body systems but is most abundant in tissues of the CNS. Approximately 70 percent of people with this disorder produce an immune protein called an "antibody" that attaches (binds) to the AQP4. Antibodies normally bind to specific foreign particles and germs, marking them for destruction, but the antibody in people with NMO attacks a normal human protein; this type of antibody is called an "autoantibody." The autoantibody in this condition is called "NMO-IgG" or "anti-AQP4."

The binding of the NMO-IgG autoantibody to the AQP4 turns on (activates) the complement system, which is a group of immune system proteins that work together to destroy pathogens, trigger inflammation, and remove debris from cells and tissues. Complement activation leads to the inflammation of the optic nerve and spinal cord, which is characteristic of NMO, resulting in the signs and symptoms of the condition.

The levels of the NMO-IgG autoantibody are high during episodes of NMO, and the levels decrease between episodes with treatment of the disorder. However, it is unclear what triggers episodes to begin or end.

TYPES OF NEUROMYELITIS OPTICA

There are two forms of NMO, the relapsing form and the monophasic form. The relapsing form is the most common. This form is characterized by recurrent episodes of optic neuritis and transverse myelitis. These episodes can be months or years apart, and there is usually partial recovery between episodes. However, most affected individuals eventually develop permanent muscle weakness and vision impairment that persist even between episodes.

For unknown reasons, approximately nine times more women than men have the relapsing form. The monophasic form, which is less common, causes a single episode of NMO that can last several months. People with this form of the condition can also have lasting muscle weakness or paralysis and vision loss. This form affects men and women equally. The onset of either form of NMO can occur anytime from childhood to adulthood, although the condition most frequently begins in a person's forties.

FREQUENCY OF NEUROMYELITIS OPTICA

Neuromyelitis optica affects approximately 1–2 per 100,000 people worldwide. Women are affected by this condition more frequently than men.

INHERITANCE OF NEUROMYELITIS OPTICA

Neuromyelitis optica is usually not inherited. Rarely, this condition is passed through generations in families, but the inheritance pattern is unknown.[2]

TREATMENT OF NEUROMYELITIS OPTICA

There is no cure for NMO. The U.S. Food and Drug Administration (FDA) has approved three drug treatments (eculizumab, inebilizumab-cdon, and satralizumab-mwge), which can reduce the risk of relapses in adults who are anti-AQP4 antibody positive.

NMO relapses and attacks are often treated with corticosteroid drugs and plasma exchange (also called "plasmapheresis," a process used to remove harmful antibodies from the bloodstream). Immunosuppressive drugs used to prevent attacks include mycophenolate mofetil, rituximab, and azathioprine. Pain, stiffness, muscle spasms, and bladder and bowel control problems can be managed with medications and therapies.

Individuals with major disability may require physical and occupational therapy, along with social services professionals to address

---

[2] MedlinePlus, "Neuromyelitis Optica," National Institutes of Health (NIH), March 1, 2015. Available online. URL: https://medlineplus.gov/genetics/condition/neuromyelitis-optica/#inheritance. Accessed February 16, 2024.

Other Conditions Linked to Multiple Sclerosis

complex rehabilitation needs. Most individuals with NMO have an unpredictable, relapsing course of disease with attacks occurring months or years apart. Disability is cumulative, the result of each attack damaging new areas of the CNS.[3]

Section 7.3 | Transverse Myelitis

WHAT IS TRANSVERSE MYELITIS?

Transverse myelitis (TM) is a neurological disorder caused by inflammation of the spinal cord, the part of the central nervous system (CNS) that sends impulses from the brain to nerves in the body. The spinal cord also carries sensory information back to the brain.

Myelitis refers to inflammation of the spinal cord. It can damage the insulating material, called "myelin," that covers nerve cell fibers. Transverse refers to the pattern of changes in sensation—there is often a band-like sensation across the trunk of the body, with sensory changes below that area.

The segment of the spinal cord at which the damage occurs determines which parts of the body are affected. Damage at one segment will affect function at that level and below. In people with TM, myelin damage most often occurs in nerves in the upper back.

Although some people recover from TM with minor or no residual problems, the healing process may take months to years. Most people with TM have at least partial recovery, with most recovery taking place within the first three months after the attack. Other people may have permanent impairments that affect their ability to perform ordinary tasks of daily living. Some people will have only one episode of TM, but others may have a recurrence, especially if an underlying illness caused the disorder.

TM may be either acute (developing over hours to several days) or subacute (usually developing over one to four weeks). In some

---

[3] "Neuromyelitis Optica," National Institute of Neurological Disorders and Stroke (NINDS), November 28, 2023. Available online. URL: www.ninds.nih.gov/health-information/disorders/neuromyelitis-optica. Accessed March 12, 2024.

people, TM is the first symptom of an autoimmune or immune-mediated disease such as multiple sclerosis (MS) or neuromyelitis optical (NMO).

SIGNS AND SYMPTOMS OF TRANSVERSE MYELITIS
Classic features and symptoms of TM include the following:
- **Weakness of the legs and arms.** People with TM may have weakness in the legs that progresses rapidly. If the myelitis affects the upper spinal cord, it affects the arms as well. People may develop paraparesis (partial paralysis of the legs) that may progress to paraplegia (complete paralysis of the legs), requiring the person to use a wheelchair.
- **Pain.** Initial symptoms usually include lower back pain or sharp, shooting sensations that radiate down the legs or arms or around the torso.
- **Sensory alterations.** Transverse myelitis can cause paresthesias (abnormal sensations such as burning, tickling, pricking, numbness, coldness, or tingling) in the legs and sensory loss. Abnormal sensations in the torso and genital region are common.
- **Bowel and bladder dysfunction.** Common symptoms include an increased frequency or urge to use the toilet, incontinence, and constipation.

Many people also report having muscle spasms, a general feeling of discomfort, headache, fever, and loss of appetite, while some people experience respiratory problems. Other symptoms may include sexual dysfunction, depression, or anxiety caused by lifestyle changes, stress, and chronic pain.

CAUSES OF TRANSVERSE MYELITIS
The following conditions appear to cause TM:
- immune system disorders appear to play an important role in causing damage to the spinal cord. These include:
  - MS, a disorder in which immune system cells that normally protect us from viruses, bacteria, and

Other Conditions Linked to Multiple Sclerosis

unhealthy cells mistakenly attack the protective coating of myelin in the brain, optic nerves, and spinal cord
- aquaporin-4 (AQP4) autoantibody associated NMO, a disorder that affects the eye nerves and spinal cord (AQP4 is a channel on the cell membrane that lets water enter the cell and helps maintain the chemical balance so that the CNS will work correctly.)
- postinfectious or postvaccine autoimmune phenomenon, in which the body's immune system mistakenly attacks the body's own tissue while responding to the infection or, less commonly, a vaccine
- an abnormal immune response to an underlying cancer that damages the nervous system
- other antibody-mediated conditions that are still being discovered
- viral infections, including herpes viruses such as varicella zoster (the virus that causes chickenpox and shingles), herpes simplex, cytomegalovirus, and Epstein-Barr; flaviviruses such as West Nile and Zika; influenza, echovirus, hepatitis B (HepB), mumps, measles, and rubella (It is often difficult to know whether direct viral infection or a postinfectious response causes the TM.)
- bacterial infections such as syphilis, tuberculosis, actinomyces, pertussis, tetanus, diphtheria, and Lyme disease (Bacterial skin infections, middle-ear infections, *Campylobacter jejuni* gastroenteritis, and mycoplasma bacterial pneumonia have also been associated with TM.)
- fungal infections in the spinal cord, including aspergillus, blastomyces, coccidioides, and cryptococcus
- parasites, including toxoplasmosis, cysticercosis, shistosomiasis, and angtiostrongyloides
- other inflammatory disorders that can affect the spinal cord, such as sarcoidosis, systemic lupus erythematosus

(SLE), Sjögren syndrome (SS), mixed connective tissue disease, scleroderma, and Behçet syndrome
- vascular disorders such as arteriovenous malformation, dural arteriovenous fistula, intraspinal cavernous malformation, or disk embolism

The exact cause of TM and the extensive damage to the bundles of nerve fibers of the spinal cord is unknown in many cases. When doctors cannot identify a cause for the disorder, they refer to it as idiopathic, which means the cause is unknown.

WHO IS MORE LIKELY TO GET TRANSVERSE MYELITIS?

Transverse myelitis can affect people of any age, gender, or race. It does not appear to be genetic or to run in families. The disorder occurs most frequently in people who are either between ages 10 and 19 years old or between 30 and 39 years old.

DIAGNOSIS OF TRANSVERSE MYELITIS

Physicians diagnose TM by taking a medical history and performing a thorough neurological examination. These tests can indicate a diagnosis of TM and rule out or evaluate underlying causes:
- **Magnetic resonance imaging (MRI).** MRI produces a cross-sectional view or three-dimensional image of tissues, including the brain and spinal cord. A spinal MRI will almost always confirm the presence of a damaged area (also called a "lesion"), within the spinal cord, while brain MRI may provide clues to other underlying causes, especially MS.
- **Computed tomography (CT).** CT scan is a type of multidimensional x-ray that may be used to detect inflammation in the spine.
- **Blood tests.** These tests may be used to identify or rule out various disorders, including HIV infection and vitamin B_{12} deficiency. Blood is tested for the

Other Conditions Linked to Multiple Sclerosis

presence of autoantibodies (anti-AQP4, anti-myelin oligodendrocyte) and antibodies associated with cancer (paraneoplastic antibodies). The presence of autoantibodies (proteins produced by cells of the immune system) is linked to autoimmune disorders and point to a definite cause of TM.
- **Lumbar puncture and spinal fluid analysis.** Also called a "spinal tap," it can identify more protein than usual in some people with TM and an increased number of white blood cells (leukocytes) that help the body fight infections.

TREATMENT FOR TRANSVERSE MYELITIS

There is no cure for TM, but there are treatments to prevent or minimize permanent neurological problems.

Treatments are designed to address infections that may cause the disorder, reduce spinal cord inflammation, and manage and reduce symptoms.

Some of the most common initial treatments for TM are as follows:
- **Intravenous corticosteroid drugs.** These drugs may decrease swelling and inflammation in the spine and reduce immune system activity. Such drugs may include methylprednisolone or dexamethasone. These medications may also be given to reduce subsequent attacks of TM in people with underlying disorders.
- **Plasma exchange therapy (plasmapheresis).** This therapy may be used for people who do not respond well to intravenous steroids. Plasmapheresis is a procedure that reduces immune system activity by removing plasma (the fluid in which blood cells and antibodies are suspended) and replacing it with special fluids, thus removing the antibodies and other proteins thought to be causing the inflammatory reaction.

- **Intravenous immunoglobulin (IVIG).** IVIG is a treatment that can help to reset the immune system. IVIG is a highly concentrated injection of antibodies pooled from many healthy donors. It can bind to the antibodies that may cause TM and remove them from circulation.
- **Pain medicines.** Medicines to reduce muscle pain include acetaminophen, ibuprofen, and naproxen. Nerve pain may be treated with certain antidepressant drugs (such as duloxetine), muscle relaxants (such as baclofen, tizanidine, or cyclobenzaprine), and anticonvulsant drugs (such as gabapentin or pregabalin).
- **Antiviral medications.** These medications may help people who have a viral infection of the spinal cord.
- **Medications.** These can also treat other symptoms and complications, including incontinence, painful muscle contractions called "tonic spasms," stiffness, sexual dysfunction, and depression.

Following initial therapy, it is critical to keep the person's body functioning during the recovery period. In rare cases when breathing is significantly affected, the person may be placed on a respirator.

Immunosuppressant treatments are used for NMO spectrum disorder and recurrent episodes of TM that are not caused by MS. They are aimed at preventing future myelitis attacks (or immune attacks on other parts of the body), and they may include steroid-sparing drugs such as mycophenolate mofetil, azathioprine, and rituximab.

Rehabilitation and Long-Term Therapy

Many forms of long-term rehabilitation are available for people who have disabilities resulting from TM. Strength and functioning may improve with rehabilitation services, even years after the initial episode.

Other Conditions Linked to Multiple Sclerosis

Although rehabilitation cannot reverse the physical damage resulting from TM, it can help people, even those with severe paralysis, become as functionally independent as possible and attain the best possible quality of life (QOL).[4]

---

[4] "Transverse Myelitis," National Institute of Neurological Disorders and Stroke (NINDS), November 28, 2023. Available online. URL: www.ninds.nih.gov/health-information/disorders/transverse-myelitis. Accessed February 16, 2024.

Chapter 8 | NIH Study on Severe Multiple Sclerosis Risk

Multiple sclerosis (MS) affects more than 2 million people worldwide. The disease happens when the body's immune system attacks the protective coating around nerve cells in the brain and spinal cord.

In a recent study, the National Institutes of Health (NIH) researchers followed 192 people with MS for seven years. They found that more than half of the patients had one or more dark-rimmed spots inside their brains. These spots may be markers for a more serious form of the disease.

Some early symptoms of MS include problems with seeing, balance, and muscle strength. But more aggressive forms have symptoms such as paralysis and serious problems with thinking and memory.

That is why researchers at the NIH and researchers around the country are working hard to help detect the disease early.

The new study was conducted with patients at the NIH Clinical Center, the largest research hospital in the United States. There, NIH researchers led by Daniel S. Reich, MD, PhD, used a powerful magnetic resonance imaging (MRI) scanner to take pictures of the brains of patients with MS.

His team then used a three-dimensional printer to compare the dark-rimmed spots in the scans with similar spots seen in brain tissue samples. They found that patients with four or more of these spots were more likely to have the aggressive form of MS than those without them.

"Our results point the way toward using specialized brain scans to predict who is at risk of developing progressive MS," Dr. Reich says.

His team previously published instructions for clinics on reprogramming their lower-powered MRI scanners to better detect these spots. The team hopes that researchers around the world will use these instructions to develop better diagnostic and treatment strategies for people with MS.[1]

TREATMENT CAN DELAY FUTURE ATTACKS

Most of the time, MS starts mildly, with unpredictable symptoms that can seem baffling. Without treatment, the disease can worsen to the point that you cannot write, speak, or walk. MS starts when the body's immune system slowly attacks the fatty coating around nerves. Without an intact coating, communication between nerves and the brain becomes impaired. However, it may be years before the first symptoms appear. The symptoms depend on which parts of the brain and spinal cord are affected. A typical symptom is blurry vision in one eye. It may develop over a day or two. It may be painful to move the eye. Or, you may have double vision. Another typical symptom is not being able to move or feel a leg. These symptoms, also known as "MS attacks," may last for days or weeks. Most people will have one attack that resolves over time. Later, they might have other attacks.

MS is usually diagnosed when people are young adults. But it can be diagnosed at any age. No one knows exactly how many people have MS. In the United States, at least 400,000 people do. It can be detected with an MRI scan of the brain and spinal cord. Areas where the immune system has attacked the coating around nerves will show up on an MRI scan. It is a complex disease. Nobody knows why it started. If you have a family history, your chance of developing MS may be greater.

---

[1] MedlinePlus, "New NIH Study May Help Predict Those at Risk for Severe MS," National Institutes of Health (NIH), January 8, 2020. Available online. URL: https://magazine.medlineplus.gov/article/new-nih-study-may-help-predict-those-at-risk-for-severe-ms. Accessed February 16, 2024.

NIH Study on Severe Multiple Sclerosis Risk

"We know that genes play a major role," says Dr. Daniel S. Reich. Research shows that hundreds of genes are involved. Most of these genes are related to the immune system and the inflammation it drives.

Researchers have noticed that your chance of developing MS may be lower if you do not smoke and you maintain a healthy weight. They have also found that people who have not been infected with a common virus known as "Epstein-Barr virus" (EBV) seem to be at lower risk of developing MS. But researchers do not know why. People who live near the equator seem at lower risk too. Researchers believe that it may be because there is more consistent sunlight there, which helps the body make vitamin D. Vitamin D may help the immune system work better and protect against MS.[2]

---

[2] *NIH News in Health,* "Managing Multiple Sclerosis," National Institutes of Health (NIH), January 2019. Available online. URL: https://newsinhealth.nih.gov/2019/01/managing-multiple-sclerosis. Accessed April 24, 2024.

Chapter 9 | Preventing Multiple Sclerosis in Children

Pediatric multiple sclerosis (MS) is a rare type of MS that affects children and teenagers. It is characterized by episodes of symptoms related to damage of the central nervous system (CNS), which is responsible for controlling the body's movements and sensations. These symptoms are caused by inflammation and damage to the protective coating around the nerves, called "myelin." Pediatric MS patients usually experience episodes of symptoms that come and go, with the first episode often involving problems with vision, movement, or feeling. Doctors can diagnose pediatric MS by looking for signs of inflammation and damage in the brain and spinal cord using MRI scans.[1]

Based on what we know so far, MS is not an inherited disease. This means that it is not passed down from parents to children. However, the genetic factors that contribute to MS are complex. If you have MS, your children may be more likely to develop MS later in life compared to a child whose parents do not have MS.

In general, a person's risk of developing MS is about 1 in 750–1,000. In identical twins, if one twin has MS, then the identical twin's risk of developing MS increases to one in four, which is significantly higher than that of the general population. In first-degree relatives, for example, the children, siblings, or parents of someone

---

[1] Genetic and Rare Diseases Information Center (GARD), "Pediatric Multiple Sclerosis," National Center for Advancing Translational Sciences (NCATS), February 2024. Available online. URL: https://rarediseases.info.nih.gov/diseases/10443/pediatric-multiple-sclerosis. Accessed April 24, 2024.

with MS, the risk of developing MS is higher than that for the general population. One study estimated this risk to be 1 in 35, which is still much lower than the risk for identical twins.

While we cannot change someone's genetic risk for developing MS, there are several environmental factors within somebody's control that may lower their risk for MS. These factors may be important to discuss with your children if you have MS.

SMOKING

Smoking is not only linked to more severe MS and a faster decline in disability, but it has also been shown to increase a person's risk of getting MS in the first place. Avoiding smoking is one of the best things someone could do to prevent MS. The good news for current smokers with MS is that stopping smoking is also linked with slowing down disability progression.

VITAMIN D

Low vitamin D levels may also play a role in increasing someone's risk for developing MS. Sun exposure is a natural source of vitamin D and decreased exposure to the sun may help explain why more people who live in northern regions have MS compared to people who live closer to the equator.

Some studies have shown that children born in an area with high rates of MS who then move, before age 15, to an area with low rates of MS adopt the risk of their new location. This suggests that early life environmental factors may play an important role in someone's later life risk for developing MS. While these factors may include vitamin D levels, more studies are needed in these areas.

OBESITY

Obesity in childhood and adolescence, especially in girls, is associated with an increased risk of getting MS later in life. Since obesity is often preventable and treatable, it is important to discuss this with children who may already be more likely to get MS to possibly lower their risk of getting MS.

Preventing Multiple Sclerosis in Children

In summary, while you may not be able to change your children's genetic risk for getting MS, it is important to know that avoiding smoking and obesity and getting enough vitamin D may help reduce their risk for developing MS later in life.[2]

---

[2] "How to Decrease Your Children's Risk for Multiple Sclerosis If You Have Multiple Sclerosis," U.S. Department of Veterans Affairs (VA), November 16, 2021. Available online. URL: www.va.gov/MS/Veterans/about_MS/How_to_Decrease_Your_Children_s_Risk_for_MS_If_You_Have_Multiple_Sclerosis.asp. Accessed February 16, 2024.

Chapter 10 | Managing Multiple Sclerosis Relapses

Multiple sclerosis (MS) is the most common disabling neurological disease of young adults with symptom onset generally occurring between the ages of 20 and 40 years. MS is a chronic disease that affects people differently. A small number of people with MS will have a mild course with little to no disability, whereas others will have a steadily worsening disease that leads to increased disability over time. Most people with MS, however, will have short periods of symptoms followed by long stretches of relative quiescence (inactivity or dormancy), with partial or full recovery. The disease is rarely fatal and most people with MS have a normal life expectancy.

The natural course of MS is different for each person, which makes it difficult to predict. The onset and duration of MS symptoms usually depend on the specific type but may begin over a few days and go away quickly or develop more slowly and gradually over many years.[1]

By its very name, multiple sclerosis tells us that there are many (multiple) scars (sclerosis) in the brain, spinal cord, and optic nerves. At the time these scars (also called "plaques") are formed, they might cause symptoms. New plaque formation accompanied by new symptoms is called a "clinical relapse," "attack," or "exacerbation." Depending on where the plaques form, they can cause

---

[1] "Multiple Sclerosis," National Institute of Neurological Disorders and Stroke (NINDS), November 28, 2023. Available online. URL: www.ninds.nih.gov/health-information/disorders/multiple-sclerosis. Accessed April 30, 2024.

different symptoms, such as vision loss, weakness, sensory changes, balance problems, double vision, slurred speech, or bladder problems. Other times new plaques do not cause any symptoms and can only be detected by magnetic resonance imaging (MRI). These kinds of events are called "radiographic relapses."[2]

STEROID RELAPSES

Relapses are new or worsening symptoms caused by MS. They can lead to a temporary or permanent increase in disability. Until recently, high doses of intravenous methylprednisolone, a type of steroid, were the standard treatment for relapses in MS. Steroids are thought to work in MS relapse due to their ability to change the immune system. Steroids may help to reduce the active inflammation seen in MS attacks by preventing the movement of immune cells from the body's circulation to the brain and spinal cord areas.

Intravenous (IV) steroids, or steroids administered via a needle placed in the vein, were found to hasten recovery after an MS attack in several placebo-controlled studies. The largest of these clinical trials was the Optic Neuritis Treatment Trial (ONTT) in 1994, which evaluated people with a first episode of optic neuritis, or inflammation of the optic nerve, a typical relapse in people with MS. In the ONTT, subjects were treated with either three days of IV methylprednisolone at a dose of 1 gm per day or low-dose oral steroids at a dose of 1 mg of prednisone per kg of body weight for 14 days. This study suggested that subjects receiving this low dose of oral steroids recovered more slowly than those treated with the high dose of IV steroids. Moreover, the study indicated that frequency of relapse was higher in the low dose oral steroid-treated group than those treated with high dose IV steroids.

The ONTT had its limitations, however. The doses of oral steroids were much lower than the doses of IV steroids. Also, subjects with optic neuritis, but not necessarily a diagnosis of MS, were included in the study. Other studies comparing oral and IV steroids

---

[2] "Multiple Sclerosis Relapses: What They Are and What to Do," U.S. Department of Veterans Affairs (VA), February 13, 2024. Available online. URL: www.va.gov/MS/TREATING_MS/MS_Relapses_What_They_Are_and_What_To_Do.asp. Accessed February 16, 2024.

had similar problems in design. Nevertheless, these studies provided a rationale for the preference of treatment of MS relapse with high dose IV steroids rather than oral steroids for the next 20 years.

In 2012, an expert evaluation of several studies concluded that there was not enough evidence to decide whether or not oral steroids are effective for MS relapses, particularly if high-dose oral steroids are used. In 2015, the landmark French COPOUSEP trial "cleared the air." This study of 200 people with relapsing remitting MS was designed specifically to decide if oral steroids were as effective as IV steroids. In contrast to the ONTT, a similar dose of steroids was administered either orally or intravenously within two weeks of onset of relapse symptoms. Both the subjects and examiners did not know which treatment participants received, and subjects were randomly chosen for each group.

The primary outcome studied was to see if disability scores one month after treatment were different between subjects treated with equivalent doses of IV versus oral steroids. Results of the trial showed that 81 percent of people in the oral group and 80 percent of people in the IV group improved at least one point in their disability score. The results confirmed that oral methylprednisolone at a dose of 1 gm/day for three days was not inferior to treatment with the same dose of IV methylprednisolone. Other outcomes examined include recovery at six months after treatment and frequency of new relapses for up to six months after treatment, which were also similar between the oral group and the IV group. Side effects for each treatment were also compared via questionnaire and were essentially the same, except for a slightly higher risk for insomnia for the oral regimen. The authors recommend taking oral steroids in the morning to avoid insomnia.

These results are very important for MS management. We now have solid evidence that the appropriate dose of steroid pills is just as effective for MS relapse as IV steroids. Advantages of pills include ease of dosing, ability to take the medication in the comfort of home, and excellent and quick availability in pharmacies of oral steroids.[3]

---

[3] "Relapse Management for Multiple Sclerosis," U.S. Department of Veterans Affairs (VA), February 13, 2024. Available online. URL: www.va.gov/MS/TREATING_MS/Relapse_Management_index.asp. Accessed April 25, 2024.

HOW DO CLINICAL RELAPSES CAUSE SYMPTOMS?

Relapse symptoms are caused by disruption of an area of the brain, spinal cord, or optic nerves due to immune cells inappropriately entering the brain and attacking the nervous tissue, a process called "neuro-inflammation." While inflammation is present, nerve cells cannot transmit signals well through the area. The signals are either completely blocked and do not reach their targets or are partly blocked and reach their targets weakly. If the blocked signal should go from the brain to the eventual target of muscles, this causes weakness. If the blocked signal should carry sensory information from the body up to the brain, this causes altered sensation such as numbness or tingling, or balance problems. With a radiographic relapse, there are no obvious symptoms because the brain and spinal cord are using alternative pathways to send their messages. However, people experiencing radiographic relapses may feel tired from the inflammation or the effort it takes to use the alternative pathways.

Clinical relapses usually last from a few days up to several months until the inflammation goes away and the damage is repaired, allowing signals in nerves to once again reach their targets. Unfortunately, repair may not be perfect, so signal conduction may not be as efficient as it was before the relapse, causing some degree of symptoms to persist.

DO ALL PEOPLE WITH MULTIPLE SCLEROSIS HAVE CLINICAL RELAPSES?

Not all people with MS have clinical relapses. About 85 percent of people with MS start off having clinical relapses followed by periods of stability. This is called "relapsing-remitting MS" (RRMS). Many of these people eventually, after 10–15 years or more, transition to secondary-progressive MS (SPMS). In SPMS, clinical relapses become less frequent and eventually stop while the ongoing MS symptoms slowly worsen over time. Some people never have clinical relapses. People with primary-progressive MS (PPMS) have MS symptoms that appear gradually and slowly worsen over time with no relapses and remissions although with some variability from day to day. People with SPMS and PPMS can get radiographic relapses, but these happen much less often than in people with RRMS.

Sometimes people with MS, particularly those with SPMS and PPMS, have sudden worsening of their MS symptoms that may seem such as a clinical relapse. However, careful searching finds that these episodes are instead actually caused by medical illnesses or emotional stresses that can temporarily worsen neurological functioning. When it is not clear if new symptoms are a relapse, an MRI can be helpful to look for new and enhancing MS plaques. This is important because new MS inflammation is generally treated very differently from another medical illness or stress causing symptoms.

WHAT SHOULD YOU DO IF YOU THINK YOU ARE HAVING A MULTIPLE SCLEROSIS RELAPSE?

First, pay attention to your symptoms. Typically, a relapse causes symptoms you never felt before or symptoms you have felt before but are now more severe than you had them in the past. Next, determine how long your symptoms are lasting; anything lasting less than 24 hours is probably not a relapse. Take note if you have other medical concerns such as urinary discomfort, cough or cold symptoms, stomach pain, skin infections, recent vaccines, or major psychological stressors in your life. This information will help your MS provider figure out what is causing the new symptoms, what additional tests might be helpful, and how best to treat you.

HOW WILL YOUR MULTIPLE SCLEROSIS HEALTH-CARE PROVIDER DETERMINE IF YOU ARE HAVING A RELAPSE?

Once you have gathered this information and your symptoms have lasted at least 24 hours, call your MS health-care provider. Depending on the severity of symptoms and other factors, your provider may require an office visit for an examination. Blood and urine testing may be ordered to see if you have an infection or other illness. An MRI may be ordered but is often not necessary. If your symptoms are severe (e.g., if you cannot walk, see, urinate, or if you have severe pain) and you cannot wait for your MS provider, see your primary care provider or visit the emergency room for evaluation. Your MS provider will determine if your symptoms are due to a clinical relapse or to a medical condition and make treatment decisions accordingly.

HOW ARE MULTIPLE SCLEROSIS CLINICAL RELAPSES TREATED?

MS clinical relapses will respond to steroid treatments. However, steroids only make the symptoms last less long, they do not affect the extent of recovery. Steroids can also have unwanted side effects, such as high blood sugar, difficulty sleeping, and anxiety or agitation. Therefore, steroids are only prescribed if symptoms are severe or disabling. When prescribed, steroids are given for three to five days, either intravenously or with pills. If relapse symptoms are mild or nondisabling, treatment may simply be rest and relaxation at home. If an underlying medical illness is found that is suspected to be causing the worsening MS symptoms, the medical problem is treated without steroid treatment. Radiographic relapses do not necessarily need steroid treatments as they are not causing disabling symptoms; however, their appearance may trigger the MS provider to switch to maintenance disease-modifying therapy. In all cases of worsening MS symptoms, regardless of their underlying causes, physical, occupational, and speech therapies may be helpful.

In summary, if you have MS and new or worsening neurological symptoms, you should suspect a clinical relapse if you have RRMS, the symptoms last for more than 24 hours, and there are no other medical or psychological stressors present. For worsening of your MS for any reason, please call your MS health-care provider to discuss your evaluation and treatment.[4]

---

[4] See footnote [1].

Managing Multiple Sclerosis Relapses

Research projects conducted by National Institute of Neurological Disorders and Stroke (NINDS) scientists or through NIH grants to universities and other sites across the United States cover a wide range of topics such as comorbidities, mechanisms of cognitive impairment, blood-brain barrier breakdown in MS, the role of sleep and circadian rhythms, rehabilitation strategies, and telehealth.[5]

---

[5] "Multiple Sclerosis," National Institute of Neurological Disorders and Stroke (NINDS), November 28, 2023. Available online. URL: www.ninds.nih.gov/health-information/disorders/multiple-sclerosis. Accessed April 30, 2024.

Part 2 | **Primary Symptoms of Multiple Sclerosis**

Chapter 11 | Fatigue

WHAT IS FATIGUE?

Fatigue can be a tremendous burden in people with multiple sclerosis (MS). It is not only the most common symptom of MS but also one of the single biggest causes of disability and decreased quality of life (QOL). To make matters worse, fatigue is one of the most difficult symptoms to communicate to others. Fatigue is a feeling, a lack of energy and motivation, an invisible symptom that cannot be detected on a brain scan, blood test, or physical exam.

CAUSES OF FATIGUE

The specific cause of fatigue in MS is not entirely clear but likely comes from multiple sources. The inflammation that causes lesions in MS can cause chemicals to be released in the brain (cytokines) that may cause fatigue. Damage to the brain's neurons likely also contributes. Neurons transmit information to the body. When damage builds up over time, this can cause impaired connections, interrupting the flow of information. Often fatigue from MS is worsened by warm weather or vigorous exercise that raises body temperature.

It is important to remember that there are also secondary causes of fatigue that are very common, results of having MS. Many symptoms of MS negatively affect sleep, which in turn makes fatigue worse. Anxiety, spasticity, pain, and urination problems can reduce the amount and quality of sleep in a person with MS. These symptoms may be modifiable with treatment.

DIAGNOSIS OF FATIGUE

If experiencing fatigue, your provider may check for other health problems that can cause fatigue, such as low thyroid hormone, sleep apnea, diabetes, anemia, and depression. Sometimes a sleep study may be helpful to make sure that you are maximizing the benefits of sleep.

TREATMENT FOR FATIGUE

There are medications that may help with fatigue for some people with MS. These should be considered, along with controlling the secondary causes of fatigue. However, the evidence that these medications work is relatively weak, and the benefit can be fairly modest. You may want to discuss with your provider whether these medications are right for you, based on consideration of potential benefits and side effects. For many, a combination of medications and other methods of treatment, such as physical therapy, exercise, and diet changes can make a big difference.

MANAGEMENT OF FATIGUE

Effective communication between the physician and patient is required to develop an individualized plan for managing a person's fatigue and overall health. Sometimes there may be difficulty expressing the significance of fatigue a person is experiencing in the setting of a brief visit with their provider when other issues may take precedence. If you are experiencing fatigue, here are a few things you can consider before talking to your provider about your fatigue.

- **Write down the most important issues.** List out the points you want to discuss with your provider to help guide your visit.
- **Journal your fatigue.** When do you have the most energy? When do you feel really drained? What activities are absolutely necessary for you to handle? Which of your activities could be delegated to others?
- **Think about your diet habits and if fatigue has influenced your eating habits.** Start with simple substitutions, such as replacing packaged snacks with nuts, seeds, or whole fruits or using beans and lentils, which provide protein without saturated fats.

Fatigue

Aim to make your plate more colorful with fruits and vegetables that provide antioxidants.
- **A brief amount of regular exercise can make a big difference.** Skilled therapists can help guide you in creating a reasonable plan and goal.
- **Discuss with your provider whether any of your medications could be causing or contributing to your fatigue.** Some medications that can cause sedation are baclofen, tizanidine, or gabapentin. Your provider may consider changing a dose or stopping a medicine if it does not seem to be helping.
- **Maximize quality of sleep through sleep hygiene.** Avoid drinking water just before bed and schedule a trip to the bathroom prior to sleeping. Avoid computer or television (TV) screens before or while you sleep. If you smoke, you should try to quit, but until you do, avoid cigarettes and alcohol in the six hours prior to bed.

Fatigue is a complex issue with no one-size-fits-all approach to solving it, but sometimes simple changes can have a big effect. The first step in getting better is taking an honest and thorough personal inventory on lifestyle changes that are feasible. The weight and challenge of swimming in the fur coat of MS-related fatigue can improve, but it often requires a multipronged treatment approach and should be coordinated with help from your primary care and MS providers.[1]

---

[1] "Multiple Sclerosis-Related Fatigue: Swimming in a Fur Coat," U.S. Department of Veterans Affairs (VA), February 15, 2022. Available online. URL: www.va.gov/MS/Veterans/symptoms_of_MS/Multiple_Sclerosis_Related_Fatigue_Swimming_in_a_Fur_Coat.asp. Accessed February 19, 2024.

Chapter 12 | Spasticity

WHAT IS SPASTICITY?

Spasticity is a common symptom of multiple sclerosis (MS). It often begins as a feeling of stiffness or muscle tightness, especially after a period of prolonged inactivity, such as a long-distance car ride or upon awakening in the morning. As a person moves around a little bit, the feeling often goes away. Eventually, though, if the stiffness is spasticity, it will likely gradually worsen until the stiffness is present most of the time.

CAUSES OF SPASTICITY

Spasticity is caused by changes in the brain or spinal cord that result from the disease process in MS. Other neurological conditions that affect the brain or spinal cord also result in spasticity, such as stroke, spinal cord injury (SCI), traumatic brain injury (TBI), or congenital conditions such as cerebral palsy (CP). These changes result in the muscles losing the smooth rhythm of normal movement that results from muscles turning on when needed and off when not needed. For example, when you bend your knee, the muscles that straighten the knee relax to allow the leg to bend easily and smoothly. And vice versa, when you straighten your knee, the muscles that bend the knee relax and allow the knee to be straightened.

COMPLICATIONS OF SPASTICITY

When spasticity gets worse, it can be associated with muscle spasms, or a bouncing or jumping in the muscles, called "clonus." Muscle spasms may occur for no apparent reason, or they may be a response to something touching a leg, for instance. Clonus is the involuntary repetitive bouncing usually most noticeable at the ankle when only the ball of the foot is on the floor. Clonus may be stopped by sliding the foot out slightly, so the heel is also in contact with the floor and, if needed, by applying firm, steady pressure onto the bent knee to help get the heel to the floor.

Spasticity can be uncomfortable, even painful, and can interfere with walking, sexuality, and self-image. Severe spasticity can cause joint contractures and deformities if left untreated.

TREATMENT FOR SPASTICITY

The first step in managing spasticity is daily stretching of affected muscles. Muscles and tendons start to lose motion at the ends of the ranges of motion first. Making sure to take each affected muscle through its full range of motion regularly is important to manage the spasticity as well as the tendency to develop deformities or contractures—permanent shortening of the tissues. For mild spasticity, stretching may be all that is needed.

For worse spasticity, there are oral medications that are readily available and widely used. The most common medication is baclofen, while the second most common medication is tizanidine. Generally, these medications are well tolerated and provide good control of spasticity. Stretching, however, must still be done to keep full range of motion when medications are used.

For people who do not tolerate the oral medications, a surgical procedure allows delivery of baclofen into the spinal canal near the spinal cord. This is called "intrathecal baclofen" delivery via a pump. The programmable pump allows a constant flow of the medication for more consistent and even management of the spasticity. The medication amount can be changed according to a person's needs throughout the day. For instance, more baclofen may be needed at night to help control spasms that cause awakening, and less may be needed during the day when you are active and moving around. Again, stretching still needs to be done with the baclofen pump.

MANAGING SPASTICITY

Often people find that doing a combination of things—stretching, changing behaviors or routines, taking medications for spasticity,

Spasticity

getting intrathecal baclofen, and/or using botulinum injections—gives them the best spasticity management.

Botulinum toxin injections, also with stretching, are used to help control severe spasms in adults' elbows, wrists, and fingers. In addition, many things can be changed in daily routines and environments to help keep spasticity from interfering. For example, if spasticity makes walking long distances difficult, a scooter may keep you moving. Systems to transport scooters are available that attach to many different types of vehicles.[1]

---

[1] "Spasticity: Take Control," U.S. Department of Veterans Affairs (VA), February 13, 2024. Available online. URL: www.va.gov/MS/Veterans/symptoms_of_MS/Spasticity_Take_Control.asp. Accessed February 19, 2024.

Chapter 13 | Tremors

WHAT IS TREMOR?
Tremor is a neurological condition that includes shaking or trembling movements in one or more parts of the body, most commonly affecting a person's hands. It can also occur in the arms, legs, head, vocal cords, and torso. The tremor may be constant or only happen sometimes. Tremor can occur on its own or as a result of another disorder.

Tremor is not life-threatening, but it may cause challenges and even lead to disabilities. Tremor can make daily life tasks, such as writing, typing, eating, shaving, and dressing more difficult.

SYMPTOMS OF TREMOR
Common symptoms may include the following:
- rhythmic shaking of the hands, arms, head, legs, or torso
- shaky voice
- difficulty with writing or drawing
- problems holding and controlling utensils, tools, or other items

Some tremors can be triggered by stress or strong emotion, being physically tired, or being in certain postures or making specific movements.

CAUSES OF TREMOR
Tremor is usually caused by a problem in the parts of the brain that control movements. Most types have no known genetic cause

although there are some forms that appear to be inherited and run in families.

Tremor can occur on its own or be a symptom of other neurological disorders such as Parkinson disease (PD), multiple sclerosis (MS), or stroke. Tremor sometimes can be caused by other medical conditions, including but not limited to the following:

- **Medicines.** Several drugs can cause tremors, including certain asthma medications, corticosteroids, chemotherapy, and drugs used for certain psychiatric and neurological disorders.
- **Heavy metals and other neurotoxins.** Exposure to heavy metals (such as mercury, manganese, lead, arsenic, etc.), organic solvents, or pesticides may cause tremors.
- **Caffeine.** Excessive caffeine may cause temporary tremor or make an existing tremor worse.
- **Thyroid disorder.** An overactive thyroid can cause tremors.
- **Liver or kidney failure.** Liver and kidney failure may cause damage in certain brain areas that leads to tremors or jerky movements.
- **Diabetes.** High or low blood sugar (hyperglycemia or hypoglycemia, respectively) may cause tremors or other involuntary movements.
- **Stress, anxiety, or fatigue.** These may be associated with tremors.

WHO IS MORE LIKELY TO GET TREMOR?

Tremor is most common among middle-aged and older adults although it can occur at any age. Generally, tremor occurs in men and women equally.

DIAGNOSIS OF TREMOR

To diagnose tremor, a doctor will perform a physical exam and review the person's medical history. They will perform a

neurological exam and test muscle tone and strength, reflexes, balance, and speech, and evaluate:
- whether the tremor occurs when the muscles are at rest or in action
- the location of the tremor in the body (and if it occurs on one or both sides of the body)
- the appearance of the tremor (tremor frequency and amplitude/size)

A doctor may take blood or urine samples to rule out certain contributing factors to the tremor. Diagnostic imaging may help determine if the tremor is the result of damage in the brain. An electromyogram, which measures involuntary muscle activity and muscle response to nerve stimulation, may identify muscle or nerve problems.

Additional tests can help determine any functional limitations such as difficulty with handwriting or the ability to hold a fork or cup.

TREATMENT FOR TREMOR

Although there is no cure for most forms of tremor, treatments are available to help manage symptoms. In some cases, symptoms may be mild enough that they do not need treatment. Treating any underlying health condition can sometimes cure or reduce a person's tremor.

Medications

Some medications can slow tremor. Some medications commonly used to treat tremor include the following:
- **Beta-blocking drugs.** These drugs can treat essential tremor and other types of action tremor in some people.
- **Certain antiseizure medications.** These medications can be effective to suppress essential tremor in people who do not respond to beta-blockers.

- **Tranquilizers (also known as "benzodiazepines")**. These may be prescribed to temporarily help some people with tremor. However, these medications can negatively affect sleep, concentration, and coordination and may cause physical dependence and withdrawal symptoms when stopped abruptly.
- **Dopaminergic medications.** These medications are often used to treat Parkinsonian tremors and other movement issues related to PD.
- **Anticholinergic medications.** These medications can be used to treat dystonic tremors in some people.
- **Botulinum toxin (commonly known as "Botox") injections.** These injections can be useful for dystonic head and hand tremor. It can also be used for essential tremor patients who do not respond to oral medications.

Surgery

Surgical procedures may be performed when tremor does not respond to medications or severely affects daily life.
- **Deep brain stimulation (DBS).** It is the most common form of surgical treatment of tremor. It uses surgically implanted electrodes to send high-frequency electrical signals to the thalamus, the deep structure of the brain that coordinates and controls some involuntary movements. A small pulse-generating device placed under the skin in the person's upper chest (similar to a pacemaker) sends electrical stimuli to the brain to temporarily stop tremor. DBS is currently used to treat Parkinsonian tremor, essential tremor, and dystonia.
- **Radiofrequency ablation.** It uses a radio wave to generate an electric current that disrupts nerves' signaling ability for six or more months. It is usually performed on only one side of the brain to improve tremor on the opposite side of the body.
- **Focused ultrasound.** It uses magnetic resonance imaging (MRI) to deliver high-frequency focused

ultrasound that creates a lesion in tiny areas of the brain's thalamus thought to be causing the tremors. The treatment is approved only for people whose essential tremor does not respond well to antiseizure or beta-blocking drugs.

Lifestyle Changes for Treating Tremor

Certain lifestyle changes and techniques may provide some relief for mild-to-moderate tremor.
- Physical, speech, and occupational therapy may help control tremor and adapt to daily challenges caused by the tremor.
- Eliminate or reduce caffeine.
- Assistive tools, such as special plates, spoons, or heavier utensils, can lessen tremor and make it easier to eat.
- Take medications on time.
- Talk with a doctor about stopping any medications that may be contributing to the tremor.
- Reduce stress or stressful situations that can aggravate the tremor.
- Wear clothes that make it easier to dress, such as those that use Velcro instead of buttons. Consider slip-on or no-tie shoes.
- Get enough sleep. (Some tremors worsen when a person is tired. Physical activity and exercise can help prevent fatigue and improve sleep.)[1]

---

[1] "Tremor," National Institute of Neurological Disorders and Stroke (NINDS), January 8, 2024. Available online. URL: www.ninds.nih.gov/health-information/disorders/tremor#toc-who-is-more-likely-to-get-tremor. Accessed February 20, 2024.

Chapter 14 | **Pain**

Pain is a symptom experienced by over 60 percent of people living with multiple sclerosis (MS). Pain is important because if left untreated pain affects relationships, mood, sleep, work, and the ability to have fun and generally enjoy life. Managing MS pain requires work.

KINDS OF PAIN EXPERIENCED

A lesion or a disruption of central nervous system (CNS) myelin is responsible for many MS symptoms and is one reason for the symptoms of pain. A lesion in your brain or spinal cord can cause nerves to fire in a crazy fashion resulting in pain, called "neurogenic pain." Pain may result from living with disability. Muscles, bones, or joints can be painful when stressed due to decreased mobility, long sitting, spasms, and improper use and disuse of these body parts. Then there is headache pain. People with MS seem to have more headache pain than people who do not have MS.

RECOGNIZING AND UNDERSTANDING PAIN

It is important to be able to describe your pain in detail, so your provider will know the best way of treating your pain. The most helpful way of relaying what your pain is like is to keep a journal. Neurogenic pain is either steady and continuous or intermittent and spontaneous. Steady pain is described as burning, tight, tingling, nagging, aching, or throbbing. Most describe the steady pain as burning in the legs, feet, and hands, while some describe the pain as icy. The nagging sensations of crawling bugs, water running down an arm or leg, or tingling, pins, and needles sensations can become so bothersome these are described and treated as pain.

Steady pain is often worse at night, with temperature changes, and with exercise. Steady pain is more common than intermittent or spontaneous pain. Intermittent pain is described as stabbing, electric shock-like, or searing. This pain may occur in any part of the body but often in the face (trigeminal neuralgia).

When writing in your pain journal, describe the feeling, jot down when the pain starts and ends, and where on your body the pain is located. Record what makes the pain worse, what makes it better, and what you are using to decrease the pain. For instance, are you using a complementary therapy such as acupuncture or an over-the-counter (OTC) treatment such as ibuprofen or a muscle rub.

TREATING PAIN

It is known that emotions such as anxiety, depression, anger, stress, and boredom can affect pain intensity. Lack of support, lack of sleep, and fatigue worsen the experience of pain. Recognizing the importance of general well-being means that in managing pain, your health-care provider is going to understand you as a whole person. Your physical experience of pain, your emotional responses, and your support system are considered in pain management. Your pain is then tackled with an integration of medications, interventions to relieve anxiety and depression, and strategies to enhance social support and help you become more active.

Relaxation, meditation, imagery, hypnosis, distraction, strong beliefs or faith, and biofeedback are strategies that increase the tolerance to pain. Getting involved in work or social activities, joining a support group, or even having a good laugh are techniques that can minimize pain. Interestingly to note, higher pain severity is reported by people with MS who are unemployed or homebound. Physical agents work to enhance or limit pain transmitters and include the application of heat, cold, or pressure, physical therapy, exercise, massage, acupuncture, yoga, tai chi, and transcutaneous electrical nerve stimulation (use of electric current to stimulate nerves for therapeutic purposes).

Medication treatment of neurogenic pain is aimed at changing the crazy nerve firing. Drugs used for epilepsy help make nerve cell

Pain

walls tight and stable. These also stop the wild nerve firing. Drugs for depression are used because the "feel good" neurotransmitters in your brain ease the perception of pain. The use of opioids remains controversial in MS pain management. Opioids or narcotics are considered when other agents become ineffective or not well tolerated. Narcotics may help you escape pain but can take away choice and true control over pain.

In summary, pain is a symptom that demands serious and ongoing attention, as it has a pervasive effect on daily living. MS pain management is an achievable goal that integrates behavioral, emotional, and physical strategies as well as medications. The goal of pain management is to optimize mood, sleep, and quality of life (QOL). While MS pain is yours to own, and ultimately you are the one to understand and make a difference in the pain experience, this is not something you need to do alone. Among many, your doctor, nurse, pain psychologist, physical therapist, spiritual advisor, friends, and significant other are there to help.[1]

---

[1] "The 'Ouch' of Multiple Sclerosis," U.S. Department of Veterans Affairs (VA), February 13, 2024. Available online. URL: www.va.gov/MS/Veterans/symptoms_of_MS/The_Ouch_of_Multiple_Sclerosis.asp. Accessed February 20, 2024.

Chapter 15 | Speech and Swallowing Problems

Multiple sclerosis (MS) causes damage to the central nervous system (CNS) and can cause lesions in the part of the brain responsible for controlling the vocal cords, diaphragm, soft palate, tongue, and lips. As a result, speech problems such as slurred speech, difficulty articulating, and dysphonia can arise. Difficulty swallowing, known as "dysphagia," can also be caused by MS-related neural damage. Since MS affects each person differently, the severity and duration of symptoms will vary from person to person. An individual's symptoms may change over the progression of MS as well.

Approximately 44 percent of people with MS experience impairments in speech or voice, and 33 percent of people with MS have trouble swallowing. Yet, only around 2 percent of people with MS receive speech therapy. Rehabilitative therapies and strategies can help manage symptoms to maintain independent function and improve quality of life (QOL).

SPEECH

Speech is a highly complex process that depends on finely controlled and coordinated muscles. Dysarthria, a speech disorder common in people with MS, can present with slurred speech, nasal speech, and a low or inappropriate volume. Some people with MS may have trouble with language production and thinking of words they want to say, which is called "aphasia." Speech difficulties can also occur secondary to other MS symptoms such as ataxia (poor muscle control that causes involuntary movements), dystonia (muscles contract involuntary), muscle spasms and stiffness, cognitive changes, and tremors.

For a thorough evaluation of your speech disorder, it is important to see a speech and language pathologist (SLP). They can help you develop skills and techniques to manage your speech impairment such as:

- **Exercise your speech muscles.** Your SLP can provide you with exercises that can be practiced daily to improve function and strengthen muscles that support breath control and speech production. These exercises will also promote relaxation of these muscles.
- **Practice speech techniques.** Your SLP can teach you techniques that can slow down your speech, help with your phrasing and pausing to help make speech clearer, and can demonstrate how to overarticulate words to make your speech more understandable.
- **Self-monitor your speech patterns.** Use a recording device to capture how you speak. This allows you to correct some of your speech issues by adjusting your volume or phrasing.
- **Use new devices and current technology to assist with your speech.** Devices like voice amplification, electronic aids, and other computer-assisted communication systems are readily available and easy to use. Many programs can be downloaded for free over the Internet.
- **Experiment with cognitive-linguistic compensatory strategies.** Your SLP can teach you strategies to help with word retrieval, information processing, organization, and more, to improve your communication.
- **Practice, practice, practice.** Working toward clear goals based on a thorough understanding of your speech difficulties is key. Try to practice in group settings with supportive friends and family who can provide you with feedback on your speech patterns.

Speech and Swallowing Problems

- **Consider medications.** Check with your provider about medications that can improve speech by helping affected muscles or related symptoms like dystonia or tremors.

SWALLOWING

Swallowing is a complex process that requires the muscles in the mouth and throat to work in a coordinated way. If nerve damage causes these muscles to become weak or uncoordinated, or numbness affects the areas, swallowing can become difficult. People with MS might have difficulty managing solids or liquids, feel like food gets stuck in their throat, or feel the need to cough while eating or drinking. Some people with MS may also feel like food "goes down the wrong pipe," which is called "aspiration." Around a quarter of people with MS experience diminished sense of taste, which can cause even more difficulty during mealtime.

Even though most people with MS experience fairly mild symptoms, swallowing dysfunction can cause serious issues such as dehydration, poor nutrition, and aspiration pneumonia. As a result, it is important to identify and treat swallowing difficulties to maximize the safety and efficiency of eating. To create a safe eating environment, incorporate modifications and routines such as:

- **Maintain oral health.** Brush your teeth and tongue thoroughly twice a day to reduce bacteria in your mouth and decrease your risk of aspiration pneumonia.
- **Sit upright when eating or drinking.** Keep your chin parallel with the table, unless instructed by a professional to do otherwise.
- **Take smaller bites of food, one at a time.** Eat slowly, and sip drinks, do not gulp.
- **Double swallows might be needed.** Double swallows refers to swallowing once to send liquids or food down, then doing a dry swallow to clear any leftover particles.
- **Post-swallowing recommendation.** It might be recommended that, after you swallow, you clear your throat and swallow again.

- **Add moisture/liquid to foods.** Foods with moisture are easier to swallow. You can also try alternating between bites of food and sips of liquid.
- **Eat smaller portions.** If you are experiencing fatigue, which can interfere with swallowing, try to consume smaller meals throughout the day instead of one or two large meals.
- **If you feel like you are getting tired while eating, take a break.** It is better to have smaller meals more frequently than a few large meals that cause fatigue.
- **Etiquette reminder.** Eat meals in a quiet environment and try not to speak when food is in your mouth.
- **If swallowing problems persist, consider seeing a speech pathologist.** They can evaluate your swallow with special imaging, such as modified barium swallow studies, to recommend targeted treatment strategies, dietary changes, or exercises.

Optimal MS management includes a multidisciplinary healthcare team focused on treating a person's unique profile of symptoms, including speech and swallowing difficulties. This team includes the person with MS and their support systems who provide essential feedback to providers as to what is working in the home environment and when modifications are needed to address these problems.

Speech and swallowing deficits can limit your QOL, but managing the symptoms with the help of an SLP can increase your ability to communicate with others, function effectively, and eat and drink safely. It is important to have a SLP complete a full evaluation so specific treatment recommendations can be made. Check with your provider about VA services that can help improve your speech and swallowing.[1]

---

[1] "Speech and Swallowing," U.S. Department of Veterans Affairs (VA), February 13, 2024. Available online. URL: www.va.gov/MS/Veterans/symptoms_of_MS/Speech_and_Swallowing.asp. Accessed April 24, 2024.

Speech and Swallowing Problems

SPEAKING

Just as the muscles involved in swallowing can be affected by MS, the muscles involved in speaking can, too. Speech difficulties, called "dysarthria," are relatively common for people with MS, with about 40–50 percent of individuals reporting changes in their communication. Speech difficulties might include slurred-sounding speech, increased fatigue with conversation, or reduced vocal loudness. This is often mild and may not affect overall intelligibility or successful communication but can be of concern to the individual. Some general strategies to support effective communication include the following:

- breath support and diaphragmatic or "belly" breathing
- increased speaking loudness
- reduced speech rate
- exaggerated articulation of each sound

In more severe case of MS, speech supplementation or speech-generating devices might be necessary. When dysarthria interferes with safety, functional communication of daily needs/desires, or general QOL, both low-tech and high-tech devices may be useful. Low-tech devices include alphabet and eye gaze boards, pictures, notebooks, or whiteboards, bells and buzzers, and simple yes/no systems. High-tech alternatives include voice amplifiers, text-to-speech devices, and applications ("apps") that can be found on smartphones and tablets.[2]

---

[2] "Swallowing, Speaking, and Thinking," U.S. Department of Veterans Affairs (VA), February 13, 2024. Available online. URL: www.va.gov/MS/Veterans/symptoms_of_MS/Swallowing_Speaking_and_Thinking.asp. Accessed February 20, 2024.

Chapter 16 | Vocal Fold Paralysis

The vocal folds are two elastic bands of muscle tissue located in the larynx (voice box) directly above the trachea (windpipe). When you breathe, your vocal folds remain apart and when you swallow, they are tightly closed. When you use your voice, however, air from the lungs causes your vocal folds to vibrate between open and closed positions.

WHAT IS VOCAL FOLD PARALYSIS?

Vocal fold paralysis (also known as "vocal cord paralysis") is a voice disorder that occurs when one or both of the vocal folds do not open or close properly. Single vocal fold paralysis is a common disorder. Paralysis of both vocal folds is rare and can be life-threatening.

If you have vocal fold paralysis, the paralyzed fold or folds may remain open, leaving the air passages and lungs unprotected. You could have difficulty swallowing, or food or liquids could accidentally enter the trachea and lungs, causing serious health problems.

WHAT CAUSES VOCAL FOLD PARALYSIS?

Vocal fold paralysis may be caused by injury to the head, neck, or chest; lung or thyroid cancer; tumors of the skull base, neck, or chest; or infection (e.g., Lyme disease). People with certain neurologic conditions, such as multiple sclerosis (MS) or Parkinson disease (PD), or who have sustained a stroke, may experience vocal fold paralysis. In many cases, however, the cause is unknown.

WHAT ARE THE SYMPTOMS OF VOCAL FOLD PARALYSIS?
Symptoms of vocal fold paralysis include changes in the voice, such as hoarseness or a breathy voice; difficulties with breathing, such as shortness of breath or noisy breathing; and swallowing problems, such as choking or coughing when you eat because food is accidentally entering the windpipe instead of the esophagus (the muscular tube that connects the throat to the stomach). Changes in voice quality, such as loss of volume or pitch, also may occur. Damage to both vocal folds, although rare, usually causes serious problems with breathing.

HOW IS VOCAL FOLD PARALYSIS DIAGNOSED?
Vocal fold paralysis is usually diagnosed by an otolaryngologist—a doctor who specializes in ear, nose, and throat disorders. He or she will ask you about your symptoms and when the problems began in order to help determine their cause. The otolaryngologist will also listen to your voice to identify breathiness or hoarseness. Using an endoscope—a tube with a light at the end—your doctor will look directly into the throat at the vocal folds. Some doctors also use a procedure called "laryngeal electromyography," which measures the electrical impulses of the nerves in the larynx, to better understand the areas of paralysis.

HOW IS VOCAL FOLD PARALYSIS TREATED?
The most common treatments for vocal fold paralysis are voice therapy and surgery. Some people's voices will naturally recover sometime during the first year after diagnosis, which is why doctors often delay surgery for at least a year. During this time, your doctor will likely refer you to a speech-language pathologist (SLP) for voice therapy, which may involve exercises to strengthen the vocal folds or improve breath control while speaking. You might also learn how to use your voice differently, for example, by speaking more slowly or opening your mouth wider when you speak. Several surgical procedures are available, depending on whether one or both of your vocal folds are paralyzed. The most common procedures change the position of the vocal fold. These may involve inserting

Vocal Fold Paralysis

a structural implant or stitches to reposition the laryngeal cartilage and bring the vocal folds closer together. These procedures usually result in a stronger voice. Surgery is followed by additional voice therapy to help fine-tune the voice.

When both vocal folds are paralyzed, a tracheotomy may be required to help breathing. In a tracheotomy, an incision is made in the front of the neck and a breathing tube is inserted through an opening, called a "stoma," into the trachea. Rather than occurring through the nose and mouth, breathing now happens through the tube. Following surgery, therapy with an SLP helps you learn how to use the voice and how to properly care for the breathing tube.[1]

---

[1] "Vocal Fold Paralysis," National Institute on Deafness and Other Communication Disorders (NIDCD), March 6, 2017. Available online. URL: www.nidcd.nih.gov/health/vocal-fold-paralysis. Accessed February 20, 2024.

Chapter 17 | Optic Neuritis

Vision is very important in almost everything we do, including watching television, reading a book, driving, and many other activities. When multiple sclerosis (MS) disturbs vision, it can have a significant consequence on quality of life (QOL). People with MS can have many different kinds of vision problems, one of the most common being optic neuritis.

WHAT IS OPTIC NEURITIS?
Optic neuritis is an inflammation or demyelination of the optic nerve, the nerve that connects the eye to the brain.

SIGNS AND SYMPTOMS OF OPTIC NEURITIS
People with optic neuritis generally complain of blurry vision or hazy vision affecting one eye. Often the center of vision is most affected, making it difficult to see people's faces or creating a "line" in the center of their vision. Some people with optic neuritis describe the blur as a "film" over their eye. Color perception is usually affected as well, with colors seeming faded or less intense in the eye affected by optic neuritis. Optic neuritis is often associated with some eye pain or discomfort, especially with eye movements, which may be described as an "ache" or "sticking sensation" behind the eye.

In optic neuritis, the blurring of vision may gradually worsen over the course of a week or so. Afterward, there is usually a gradual recovery of vision, occurring over a four- to six-week period.

WHO IS AFFECTED BY OPTIC NEURITIS?

More than half of all people with MS will experience optic neuritis at some point in their lives. In fact, for 15–20 percent of people with MS, optic neuritis will be the first sign of the disease. Not all people who get optic neuritis, however, will go on to develop MS. Many studies have examined this relationship between optic neuritis and MS over time. Depending on the study, the risk of developing MS after an episode of optic neuritis varies 42–63 percent—roughly 50/50 odds.

DIAGNOSIS OF OPTIC NEURITIS

Though optic neuritis generally goes away on its own, with or without treatment, it is still important for people with optic neuritis to be seen by a neurologist to find out if MS is likely or not. For people who already have a diagnosis of MS, it may still be important to see a neurologist after an episode of optic neuritis to review MS treatment options.

TREATMENT FOR OPTIC NEURITIS

Intravenous (IV) methylprednisolone (a type of steroid known as "Solu-Medrol®") is often given to treat optic neuritis. IV steroids do not appear to improve the ultimate visual outcome, but they do seem to speed up the recovery of vision. With or without steroid treatment, optic neuritis almost always gets better, though the vision in the affected eye may not return 100 percent. Vision in the optic neuritis eye might not be as clear as before, and colors may remain faded or "washed out." Depth perception or three-dimensional (3D) vision is often not as good after an episode of optic neuritis, making it more difficult to judge distances, as when climbing stairs or reaching for objects.

Brain magnetic resonance imaging (MRI) can be very useful in predicting which person with optic neuritis will go on to develop MS. People with optic neuritis who have a normal brain MRI have a relatively low risk of going on to develop MS, ranging 8–25 percent, depending on the study. People with optic neuritis who have demyelination (also called "spots," "plaques," or "lesions") on their

Optic Neuritis

brain MRI, have a much higher risk of developing MS, possibly as high as 80 percent.

Though this risk is significant, and much greater than the risk of MS in people who start out with a normal brain MRI, it should be noted that 20–40 percent of the "high-risk" people in these studies who had an episode of optic neuritis did not go on to develop MS even after many years of follow-up.[1]

---

[1] "Optic Neuritis," U.S. Department of Veterans Affairs (VA), February 15, 2022. Available online. URL: www.va.gov/MS/Veterans/symptoms_of_MS/Optic_Neuritis.asp. Accessed February 20, 2024.

Chapter 18 | **Poor Balance**

Multiple sclerosis (MS) affects different parts of the brain or spinal cord in different people, causing somewhat different problems for each person. Many people with MS have poor balance and are at risk for falling. Research is helping scientists find out why this happens and how to help people with MS fall less often.

SIGNS AND SYMPTOMS OF IMBALANCE

Imbalance is one of the most common symptoms of MS. People with MS often say they feel off balance and researchers have found three main types of balance problems in people with MS. First, when people with MS stand still, they sway more than people without MS. They also increase this swaying more than expected when they close their eyes or reduce their base of support by standing on one leg or with their feet together. Second, when leaning, reaching, or stepping, people with MS cannot go as far or move as quickly as people without MS. Third, people with MS have difficulty maintaining their balance if they are pushed or pulled.

COMPLICATIONS OF IMBALANCE

Imbalance can lead to falls. People with MS fall frequently and often fall badly enough to be injured. More than 50 percent of people with MS fall at least once in six months and around 30 percent fall twice or more. Some people with MS are so afraid of falling that they stop being active to avoid falls. People with MS also say they fall more if they try to pay attention to too many things at once or if they are fatigued or overheated.

TREATMENT FOR IMBALANCE

Scientists are trying to develop effective treatments to improve balance and prevent falls in people with MS. These treatments generally are not medications. The treatments include exercises, home and activity modification, education, and sometimes a device such as a brace, cane, or walker.[1]

Methylphenidate Use in Multiple Sclerosis

Many physicians prescribe the drug methylphenidate to their patients with MS to relieve fatigue or improve balance and gait in their patients with MS. A study by researchers with the VA Portland Health Care System and the Oregon Health Science University looked at 24 persons with MS between the ages of 20 to 65 with poor balance and walking difficulties. Half received a placebo, and the others received escalating doses of methylphenidate over a six-week period.

The researchers found that while average performance in tests of walking, balance, and fatigue improved in both groups, greater improvements were found in those receiving placebo than any dose of methylphenidate. They also calculated a 60 percent probability of harmful effects of methylphenidate at any dose, compared to placebo.[2]

LIFESTYLE MODIFICATIONS FOR MANAGING IMBALANCE

Exercising in a standing position with gradually increasing balance challenges, such as tai chi, can be particularly helpful for improving balance. Modifications to prevent falls include minimizing distractions while walking and removing hazards. Avoid standing or walking when doing difficult mental tasks. Go to the store at less busy times and remove rugs and cords you could trip over at home. Education about fall risk will help you make good decisions.

---

[1] "Staying Upright: Avoiding Falls," U.S. Department of Veterans Affairs (VA), February 13, 2024. Available online. URL: www.va.gov/MS/Veterans/symptoms_of_MS/Staying_Upright_Avoiding_Falls.asp. Accessed February 20, 2024.

[2] "Multiple Sclerosis," U.S. Department of Veterans Affairs (VA), January 15, 2021. Available online. URL: www.research.va.gov/topics/multiple_sclerosis.cfm. Accessed April 25, 2024.

Poor Balance

And, using a cane or hiking poles, well-fitting shoes, and/or a leg brace may give you the extra support you need to stay safe and avoid falling.

More research is needed to know what works best, but for now, people with MS should get help from their doctor and a physical therapist to choose the strategies most likely to improve their balance and reduce their risk of falling.[3]

---

[3] See footnote [1].

Chapter 19 | Bladder Dysfunctions

Changes in bladder function are common after developing multiple sclerosis (MS), and they often occur early in the disease process. Between 50 and 90 percent of people with MS will develop bladder problems at some point. The big question is, why does this occur?

The symptoms of bladder problems are wide-ranging and can include the following:
- **Urgency.** Barely getting to the bathroom in a timely manner.
- **Frequency.** Feeling the need to urinate more than every two to three hours.
- **Hesitancy.** Being unable to easily start the flow of urine.
- **Incontinence.** A loss of control of urine.
- **Nocturia.** Being awakened from a restful state by a need to urinate.
- **Double voiding.** Needing to urinate again a few minutes after voiding.

Other symptoms can be felt, such as the bladder not being empty after urinating, involuntary leaking of urine, difficult or painful discharge of urine, and urinary tract infections (UTIs).

Bladder symptoms are broken down into three basic types of problems: emptying problems (hypoactive bladder), storage problems (hyperactive bladder), and a mixture of these two types of problems (combined dysfunction). Each of these types of problems has a different treatment approach.

HYPOACTIVE BLADDER

Approximately 20 percent of people with MS have a hypoactive bladder. A hypoactive bladder overfills and stretches the bladder wall, causing the sensors that trigger bladder contractions to stop working. Additionally, often the sphincter that allows urine to leave the bladder does not release and the urge to urinate does not occur until after a large volume of urine has collected (and sometimes not at all!). The danger with this type of bladder is that when it becomes overfilled, urine can back up into the kidneys, causing kidney damage or infection.

The methods used to treat this condition are abdominal tapping (tapping on your lower abdomen to trigger a urination reflex), double voiding, adequate fluid intake, good bowel management, catheterization (intermittent catheterization or indwelling Foley/suprapubic urinary catheter), and, for males, good prostate care. Medications, such as bethanechol, to stimulate bladder contractions or reduce prostate swelling with prostate or antihypertensive medications have been successfully used.

HYPERACTIVE BLADDER

The majority of people with MS (60%) have the opposite type of bladder—a hyperactive bladder. A hyperactive bladder does not hold the normal amount of urine before the urge to urinate occurs. Instead of triggering urination when it fills to 350–400 ml (normal), the urge occurs at 150–200 ml (or less), making it important to always know where every bathroom is located.

Treatments for this type of problem include decreasing irritants that trigger bladder spasms (caffeine, artificial sweeteners, alcohol, tobacco, and spicy foods), reducing excessive weight, practicing good bowel care (to reduce the amount of abdominal pressure on the bladder), pelvic muscle exercises (especially with women), and learning to manage when and where urination occurs.

Managing urine output can involve a number of strategies: wearing easily and quickly opened/removed lower garments, the use of external urinary drainage devices or protective pads/garments and determining what the best time and amount of fluid intake should

Bladder Dysfunctions

be. Changing the volume or time fluids are consumed will help make sure the need to urinate does not occur at inopportune times.

The last common treatment strategy is the use of medications. Common medications used include antispasmodics (such as baclofen), bladder relaxing medications (such as oxybutynin and tolterodine), or botulinum toxin (Botox) injections into the bladder sphincter.

COMBINED DYSFUNCTION

The third type of problem is a mixture of these first two problems and may be more difficult to treat. With this type of bladder dysfunction, the bladder wall spasms, but the sphincter releasing urine will not relax and open. Finding the correct balance of the above treatments that work best can be a trial-and-error process. Most people are able to find a combination of treatment strategies that work well for them by working with their health-care provider.[1]

---

[1] "Bladder Changes in Multiple Sclerosis," U.S. Department of Veterans Affairs (VA), February 13, 2024. Available online. URL: www.va.gov/MS/Veterans/symptoms_of_MS/Bladder_Changes_in_Multiple_Sclerosis.asp. Accessed February 20, 2024.

Chapter 20 | Cognitive Deficits

Cognition is a fancy word to refer to thinking processes, such as attention, memory and learning, or executive functions (think planning, organizing, goal setting, and time management). Some individuals with multiple sclerosis (MS) report changes in cognition, which may include the following:
- increased reliance on organizational systems, such as day planners, smartphones, or alarms
- more difficulty making decisions
- reduced ease of remembering names, places, conversations, or recent events
- more difficulty "multitasking," tuning out distractions, or focusing for a long period of time
- problems with word-finding
- slowed information processing

Typically, these changes do not affect an individual's overall ability to function independently but may require more support and strategies, including use of sticky notes, maps or global positioning system (GPS) devices, day planners or smartphones, or requests for repetition or for written information.[1]

Research studies on cognitive function in MS have demonstrated that as many as 50–66 percent of people will experience some cognitive changes over the course of the disease. Even though

---

[1] "Swallowing, Speaking, and Thinking," U.S. Department of Veterans Affairs (VA), February 13, 2024. Available online. URL: www.va.gov/MS/Veterans/symptoms_of_MS/Swallowing_Speaking_and_Thinking.asp. Accessed February 20, 2024.

the severity of these changes can vary from mild to quite severe, the majority of these changes are in the mild-to-moderate range. It is important to familiarize yourself with the kinds of changes that can occur:

- **Cognitive changes can occur at any time, and their severity does not appear to correlate with either length of time since diagnosis or the level of a person's physical disability.** For example, a person with significant physical limitations, who has had MS for some time, can be totally free of cognitive symptoms, while a person with a recent diagnosis and few physical symptoms can have significant cognitive impairment.
- **Even relatively mild symptoms can have a pretty big effect on various activities of daily living.** For instance, people with MS are more likely to leave the workforce because of cognitive symptoms and fatigue than because of mobility problems. Early departure from the workforce is a critical issue for people with MS, but it can often be avoided with adequate symptom management.
- **Cognitive fatigue can interfere with your ability to get things done.** Research has shown that people with MS who are concentrating very hard on a cognitively strenuous task can experience a kind of mental fatigue that feels like acute "brain drain." Fortunately, a brief rest from the task will generally help you get back on track.
- **Cognitive changes tend to progress slowly over time.** Even though MS relapses can include a sudden worsening of cognitive symptoms as well as physical ones, which tend to improve as a relapse ends, problems with thinking and memory do not generally disappear completely.
- **The sooner these kinds of cognitive problems are identified, the easier it is to develop effective strategies to manage them.** Small problems are always easier to work around than bigger ones. When you are able to put your finger on a problem with thinking or

Cognitive Deficits

memory early on, you can find ways to compensate for it before the problem begins to interfere significantly with your daily life.

Like the physical symptoms that can occur in MS, the cognitive changes are highly variable from one person to another. One person may experience a lot of problems while another person experiences none or very few. In other words, no two people experience the same changes in exactly the same way. However, the following types of problems are the most common in MS. There are several types of cognitive problems.

MEMORY

Historically, experts believed that the primary memory problem for people with MS was with the retrieval of information that had been stored in memory. In other words, these experts believed that a person could learn new information and tuck it away in memory but then be unable to recall or retrieve it from storage when needed. More recent evidence suggests that the problem may involve the initial learning phase. People with MS may need longer time or a few more repetitions to learn and store new information successfully. After it has been stored; however, it can generally be recalled without difficulty. For example, if you have memory problems, it may take you longer than someone without memory problems to memorize a list of words. But once you have the words memorized, you will remember them just as well as the other person does.

INFORMATION PROCESSING

Slowed processing is important because it may be the primary reason why a person with MS needs more time or repetitions to learn new information. When processing is impaired, the person has trouble keeping up with incoming information, whether it is from conversations, television (TV) shows, or books. People describe this slowing by saying, "I can still do everything I used to be able to do, but it all seems much slower—like my brain needs to be oiled."

ATTENTION AND CONCENTRATION
Attention and concentration, which form the basis for many other cognitive functions, can also be impaired by MS. For example, people who are used to being able to focus on many complex and competing tasks at the same time may notice some frustrating changes, such as being easily distracted by interruptions or competing stimuli, having difficulty moving smoothly from one task to another or finding it more difficult to multitask (an essential skill in any occupation, particularly parenthood).

EXECUTIVE FUNCTIONS
Executive functions include the high-level processes of planning, prioritizing, and problem-solving. Research has shown that people with MS may find thinking through complex problems or projects more difficult because they lose the mental agility to shift from concept to concept along the way. People often describe this impairment as "feeling stuck" or "lost in a maze."

VISUAL PERCEPTUAL SKILLS
Visual perceptual skills, which include simple perception or recognition of objects, as well as sense of direction and orientation in space, can be affected in MS. These problems can interfere with activities ranging from reading a map or driving, to programming your vestibulo-collic reflex (VCR) or dealing with those pesky "some assembly required" projects.

VERBAL FLUENCY
Verbal fluency includes the ability to find the word you are looking for quickly and easily. "It's on the tip of my tongue" is a particularly common complaint from those who have MS, as is "I'm talking to someone and all of a sudden I'm stuck without the word I need." People who experience these kinds of problems may feel less confident about their ability to talk smoothly and comfortably with others.

Cognitive Deficits

GENERAL INTELLIGENCE

People with MS sometimes say they feel "dumber." The good news is that general intelligence is usually not affected in MS. However, individual functions that make up general intelligence, such as memory, reasoning, or perceptual skills, can be affected or slowed temporarily during a relapse or more permanently over the course of the disease. So a person's intelligence quotient (IQ), which is a composite score made up of individual subtest scores on all these functions, can become lower over time.

If you are experiencing some of the cognitive problems that were outlined here, it is important for you to make an appointment with your health-care provider. Your provider can refer you to either a clinical psychologist or social worker for some testing. After your testing, the specialist can help you address some of your cognitive problems with specific cognitive retraining, memory aids and devices, and other supportive strategies to help you improve your quality of life (QOL).[2]

---

[2] "Understanding How Multiple Sclerosis Can Affect Your Cognition," U.S. Department of Veterans Affairs (VA), February 13, 2024. Available online. URL: www.va.gov/MS/Veterans/symptoms_of_MS/Understanding_How_Multiple_Sclerosis_Can_Affect_Your_Cognition.asp. Accessed February 20, 2024.

Chapter 21 | Depression

Depression is common in the general population, but depression is even more common in people with multiple sclerosis (MS). Approximately 50 percent of people with MS will experience an episode of major depression; a clinical diagnosis that requires at least two weeks with five or more depressive symptoms. Major depression is not only more common in people with MS than in the general population but also more common in people with MS than in people with other chronic diseases. Although major depression is a serious condition, remember that effective treatment is available.

WHY SHOULD SOMEONE BE CONCERNED IF THEY ARE DEPRESSED?

Depression is a serious condition, and if left untreated, can lead to chronic depression. Depression is a medical disorder that can be mild, severe, or even life-threatening. Not only it can affect a person's quality of life (QOL), but it can also interfere with relationships, jobs, and a person's overall health. People with depression are at higher risk for suicide, and the suicide rate is even higher for those with both MS and major depression. Depression is not something to ignore or "just get over." It is a disorder that requires close monitoring and treatment.

HOW CAN YOU TELL IF YOU HAVE MAJOR DEPRESSION?

The two main symptoms that may indicate major depression are persistent sadness and loss of interest in usually enjoyable activities. A person may also sleep too much or too little, eat too much or too little, feel excessively guilty, have decreased concentration, or decreased energy. Some might be irritable, angry, have feelings of hopelessness, or have thoughts of hurting themselves or others. Often, signs and symptoms of depression, such as fatigue or difficulty with concentration, can mimic symptoms of MS. Everyone feels down or overwhelmed every once in a while, but when a person feels this way for more than two weeks or is starting to have difficulty enjoying life, it is time for a more complete evaluation by a heath-care provider.

WHAT SHOULD YOU DO IF YOU THINK YOU ARE DEPRESSED?

If you think you are depressed, talk to a health-care provider. This could be your primary care team, neurologist, or rehabilitation doctor. These providers can help with diagnosing and treating depression, or they may refer you to a behavioral health specialist such as a psychiatrist or psychologist for further assessment and treatment. If a person is having thoughts of suicide, immediate attention is required: dial 988 for the national suicide and crisis lifeline.

HOW IS MAJOR DEPRESSION TREATED?

Treatment options for major depression may include antidepressant medication, counseling, lifestyle modifications, and support, as well as complementary and alternative medicine. Effective treatment often includes a combination of these therapies. There are many antidepressant medications, and some have the added benefit of treating pain, insomnia, or fatigue. For some people, treating their depression also reduces some of their MS symptoms, such as fatigue, impaired cognition, and memory difficulties. Although each person responds to medications uniquely, overall, antidepressants are well tolerated. Other substances can interfere with the effectiveness of antidepressants, and a health-care provider should be informed about all medications and supplements you are taking, as well as alcohol and drug use before starting an antidepressant. Antidepressants can take as long as six to eight weeks to work, so

Depression

do not become discouraged if results are not seen immediately. If you have depression, talk with your MS care team. Depression can be treated successfully![1]

Research suggests that people who have depression and another medical illness tend to have more severe symptoms of both illnesses. They may have more difficulty adapting to their medical condition, and they may have higher medical costs than those who do not have both depression and a medical illness. Symptoms of depression may continue even as a person's physical health improves.

A collaborative care approach that includes both mental and physical health care can improve overall health. Research has shown that treating depression and chronic illness together can help people better manage both their depression and their chronic disease.[2]

---

[1] "Questions and Answers about Depression," U.S. Department of Veterans Affairs (VA), February 13, 2024. Available online. URL: www.va.gov/MS/Veterans/symptoms_of_MS/Questions_and_Answers_About_Depression.asp. Accessed February 20, 2024.

[2] "Chronic Illness and Mental Health: Recognizing and Treating Depression," National Institute of Mental Health (NIMH), 2021. Available online. URL: www.nimh.nih.gov/health/publications/chronic-illness-mental-health. Accessed April 30, 2024.

Chapter 22 | Common Sleep Disorders

Sleep plays an important role in your physical health and well-being. Sleep supports healthy brain functioning, is involved in the healing and repair of your heart and blood vessels, regulates mood, reduces stress, and even helps your immune system defend your body against foreign or harmful substances. The average adult needs seven to nine hours of sleep each day to function well. Yet many people do not get enough sleep.

People with multiple sclerosis (MS) often say they sleep poorly at night and are fatigued in the daytime. In the general population, the three most common sleep problems reported are insomnia, sleep apnea, and restless legs syndrome (RLS). Research suggests that people with MS are even more likely to have all of these problems.

INSOMNIA

Insomnia is characterized by problems getting to sleep, problems staying asleep, or by waking up too early. Insomnia can have multiple causes and is a significant problem at some point for almost 50 percent of people with MS. Insomnia can be caused by MS symptoms that occur at night, such as pain, muscle spasms, and urinary frequency, that then disrupt sleep. Medications, including some antidepressants, selective serotonin reuptake inhibitors (SSRIs), stimulants used to treat daytime fatigue, and corticosteroids used to treat MS relapses, can also contribute to insomnia. Depression, which is common in people with MS, is also associated with insomnia.

Although occasional self-medication of insomnia with over-the-counter (OTC) sleep medications can help, if you use them often, they will probably stop working and will also make you feel sleepy or foggy during the day. Many approaches can be effective for treating insomnia, including adjusting your current medication regimen, addressing MS symptoms that are contributing to poor sleep, using nonmedication cognitive behavioral therapy (CBT) approaches and, in resistant cases, using prescribed sleep enhancing medications.

SLEEP APNEA

Sleep apnea affects at least one in five Americans and probably an even greater proportion of people with MS. Sleep apnea is characterized by repeatedly stopping breathing during sleep. These frequent pauses in breathing can cause fragmented sleep as well as low blood oxygen levels. Untreated, sleep apnea is associated with poor daytime functioning, mood, and memory problems and, if severe, cardiovascular disorders such as heart disease and stroke. Sleep apnea may also worsen fatigue, poor energy, and daytime tiredness, all of which are common in people with MS. Treatment of sleep apnea can reduce both the risks associated with sleep apnea and reduce fatigue, poor energy, and daytime tiredness.

RESTLESS LEGS SYNDROME

Restless legs syndrome is characterized by an uncomfortable urge to move your legs or, more rarely, other body areas, with the urge being temporarily relieved by moving the involved body area. RLS symptoms are generally worst in the evening or at night. RLS may affect up to one in three of individuals with MS and is three times more common in people with MS than in the general population. In people with MS, RLS is more common in those who are older, have had MS for longer, have primary progressive MS, and have greater disability. The exact cause of RLS is not known, but RLS appears to be linked with iron metabolism in the brain. Checking for low iron levels with a blood test, and replacing iron when low, can improve symptoms. Decreasing the intake of caffeine, nicotine,

Common Sleep Disorders

and alcohol, massaging your legs, and taking warm baths before bedtime may decrease RLS symptoms. When these interventions fail, medications to treat RLS symptoms are available.

Sleep problems such as insomnia, sleep apnea, and RLS are common and are more common in people with MS than in the general population. These sleep problems may be troublesome on their own and may contribute to daytime fatigue, poorer quality of life (QOL), and may be associated with greater disability. Fortunately, treatments are available for the most common sleep problems. If you have poor quality, unrefreshing sleep, discuss your symptoms with your provider, so they can initiate appropriate testing and treatment. Good sleep practices, such as keeping a regular bedtime and wake time, protecting your sleep time from other activities, setting up your bedroom only for sleep, and limiting caffeinated beverages can also help. While sleep-related symptoms may not completely resolve with treatment, most people experience substantial improvements in daytime functioning and an improved sense of well-being with treatment.[1]

---

[1] "Common Sleep Disorders and Multiple Sclerosis," U.S. Department of Veterans Affairs (VA), February 13, 2024. Available online. URL: www.va.gov/MS/Veterans/symptoms_of_MS/Common_Sleep_Disorders_and_Multiple_Sclerosis.asp. Accessed February 20, 2024.

Chapter 23 | Sexual Dysfunction

Sexual arousal begins in the brain. The brain sends messages to the sexual organs along the nerve pathway in the spinal cord. Multiple sclerosis (MS) related damage to these nerve pathways can directly or indirectly impair sexual functioning. Nerve damage can contribute to diminished sexual response and feelings. MS symptoms can get in the way of sexual initiation or satisfaction. Symptoms of fatigue can be the biggest culprit or spasms that seem to be worse at night or when lying down. Weakness contributes to exhaustion and may be a limiting factor in initiating sexual activity.

WHAT IS SEXUAL DYSFUNCTION?

Sexual dysfunction is a common symptom that affects more than 75 percent of people living with MS, more often than in people with other chronic diseases. Sexual dysfunction can present in many ways, limiting your ability to be sexual with your partner, to behave as a sexual being, and benefit from this way of expressing love and intimacy. The ability to be a sexual person is not lost because you live with MS although you may need to learn new ways to be sexual and accept things that are not in your control. Intimacy is a feeling of belonging to another, involves trust, and is both an emotional and physical sharing of one's most personal nature. Your MS does not need to interfere with your ability to be intimate.

Recognition of sexual dysfunction can help people with MS understand the problem, find treatment, build healthier relationships, enhance self-esteem, reduce depression, and improve quality of life (QOL).[1]

CAUSES OF SEXUAL DYSFUNCTION

Sexual dysfunction in MS has many causes:

Primary causes. These may be the direct result of demyelinating lesions in the central nervous system (CNS) that can affect sexual response and sexual feelings. Primary sexual dysfunction includes decreased or loss in libido, painful or uncomfortable genital sensations (burning, tingling, and numbness), and/or altered orgasmic response in both women and men. Women may experience decreased vaginal lubrication and dryness, inorgasmia, and low sex drive. Men may experience difficulty achieving and/or maintaining an erection, and diminished frequency of ejaculation.

Secondary causes. Sexual dysfunction problems arise as a consequence of disability caused by MS. Examples of secondary symptoms include poor bladder and bowel control, fatigue, muscle weakness, spasticity, immobility, tremor, cognitive impairment, and sensory problems. Secondary sexual dysfunction can also be a result of non-MS health conditions such as hypertension, diabetes, depression, hypercholesterolemia, obesity, and smoking. In addition, medications that are used for MS (spasticity, urinary frequency, and sensory pain) and non-MS diseases (hypertension, diabetes, and depression) can further contribute to secondary sexual dysfunction.

Tertiary causes. Sexual dysfunction in MS occurs as a result of disability related to psychological, social, and cultural issues that affect sexual response. These variables can include anxiety, low self-esteem, altered marital and family roles, changes in body image, and fear of rejection by one's partner.

Although sexual dysfunction is a prevalent problem and can be caused by a host of variables, for both men and women, it is a

---

[1] "That Part of You That Is Sexual," U.S. Department of Veterans Affairs (VA), February 13, 2024. Available online. URL: www.va.gov/MS/Veterans/symptoms_of_MS/That_Part_of_You_That_is_Sexual.asp. Accessed February 21, 2024.

topic that is frequently overlooked, and often left undiscussed and untreated.[2]

SEXUAL DYSFUNCTION IN WOMEN WITH MULTIPLE SCLEROSIS

For women, low desire or no desire is usually the first and foremost problem. Physical changes include lack of lubrication (dryness), genital numbness, decreased vaginal tone, and pain during intercourse. Body image is important to women, as are acceptance and personal security. Women rate affection and emotional communication as more important than orgasm. For women, a sexual partner who is tender and romantic, with touching, kissing, caressing, and extended foreplay is often ideal. Communication, honesty, warmth, and understanding are important for women.

SEXUAL DYSFUNCTION IN MEN WITH MULTIPLE SCLEROSIS

For men, sexual problems may occur with erections and ejaculation. Men often desire sexual partners who do not make demands and appreciate partners who are reassuring and supportive, without pressure regarding erections or performance. Men also want to feel secure in the relationship and share affection.

The first step in managing sexual dysfunction in MS is accepting that it is a common symptom that should, and can, be addressed. Sexual dysfunction not only affects QOL but can also contribute to relationship conflict, depression, isolation, performance anxiety, and fear of intimate relationships and sexual encounters. Talk to your provider about your symptoms and what can be done to help. Physical and occupational therapists can help with positioning, techniques, and "tools" while a mental health professional can help you address emotional issues that may be hindering intimacy.[3]

Sexual dysfunction can result from damage to nerves running through the spinal cord. Sexual problems may also stem from MS

---

[2] "Sexual Dysfunction and Multiple Sclerosis," U.S. Department of Veterans Affairs (VA), February 13, 2024. Available online. URL: www.va.gov/MS/Veterans/symptoms_of_MS/Sexual_Dysfunction_and_Multiple_Sclerosis.asp. Accessed February 21, 2024.
[3] See footnote [1].

symptoms such as fatigue, cramped or spastic muscles, and psychological factors. Some of these problems can be corrected with medications. Psychological counseling may be helpful.[4]

Men who experience erectile dysfunction should talk to their provider about the many medications in both pill and injectable form that can help. Before buying "Men's Performance Supplements," you should discuss the ingredients with your provider, so they can advise you if they are safe with your other medicines and any other medical conditions you may have. For example, yohimbine, a herbal supplement advertised to promote sexual function, may be dangerous to your liver, especially when taking some MS disease modifying treatments.

TIPS TO MANAGE SEXUAL DYSFUNCTION

Manage other MS symptoms that might get in the way of sexual satisfaction. If spasticity is a problem, time sexual activity between one and four hours after taking baclofen. If fatigue is a problem, take advantage of morning sex, which may be your time of peak energy. If you experience weakness, consider different positions to conserve energy and consider using supports (wedge, pillow, and support chair) to reduce strain or pressure on your body. Lack of bladder or bowel control can be addressed by using the lavatory immediately before sex. Genital stimulators can help compensate for decreased sensitivity. Know that alcohol, nicotine, some medications, and even some foods may diminish your sexual response.

Intimacy and closeness are important to your life satisfaction. Intimacy can be scary, even more so with fears around performance, rejection, failing to satisfy, and fear that MS symptoms will spoil a sexual encounter. Having an open and honest conversation with your partner about your fears is a good start to fuel greater intimacy. Have realistic expectations. Focus on the process rather than the goal. Plan a date night. Enjoy intimate times, such as holding hands and making eye contact. Create romance. Light candles, play music from your most romantic days, bring out that scent you

---

[4] "Multiple Sclerosis," National Institute of Neurological Disorders and Stroke (NINDS), August 1, 2020. Available online. URL: www.ninds.nih.gov/health-information/disorders/multiple-sclerosis. Accessed April 25, 2024.

Sexual Dysfunction

wore in high school, and touch yourself and your partner all over to discover what body mapping is all about. Engage in activities that have nothing to do with MS.

You are a sexual being. Having love and intimacy is a basic human need. Sex is an important aspect of love and intimacy. Be open to making changes to improve your sexual functioning. Talk to your provider and MS team about your sexual concerns. They can refer you to resources that will help.[5]

---

[5] See footnote [1].

Part 3 | Diagnostic Tests, Treatments, and Therapies for Multiple Sclerosis

Chapter 24 | Preparing for Annual Primary Care Evaluation

Staying well with multiple sclerosis (MS) depends on taking charge of your general health as well as keeping on top of your MS. Because people with MS can still have medical conditions such as high blood pressure, high cholesterol, heart disease, diabetes, and cancers, it is important to have a yearly primary care evaluation. This visit should include a comprehensive medical history review and general medical examination.

During these visits, your primary care provider can manage any health problems you may have and plan for any routine health screenings.

Primary care providers work closely with MS specialists to provide comprehensive care for you. To successfully manage your MS, it is important to be seen annually by an MS specialist as well. This is generally someone in the neurology, rehabilitation, or spinal cord injury department with additional training in MS who is capable of performing a full evaluation of your needs. This specialty evaluation should include a comprehensive neurological history review and examination.

The evaluations can be done in a single outpatient visit, multiple outpatient visits, or in some instances as an inpatient. Your MS evaluation is a great opportunity to find out what is new in the management of MS and to stay ahead of problems that limit your activities or ability to participate in society. A careful determination of whether MS is affecting other aspects of your health, and developing the best management strategy for you, will improve your health and general well-being. If you do not know your MS specialist or do not have an upcoming appointment, ask your primary care provider for a referral.

You can help prepare for an efficient, productive MS visit. Write a list of your most important questions and identify which are priorities ahead of time. As with your primary care visit, be sure to bring all medications and non-Veterans Affairs medical documentation with you to your appointment.

The following are some common questions your MS specialist may ask:
- How active has your MS been over the last year?
- Are you having any memory, speech, or cognitive difficulties?
- Are you experiencing fatigue?
- How are you sleeping?
- Are you experiencing any depression or anxiety?
- Are you experiencing any pain? If yes, where and when?
- Are you experiencing any spasticity or muscle spasms?
- Are you having any swallowing or breathing difficulties?
- Are you experiencing any bladder difficulties such as incontinence, urgency, difficulty voiding, or have you had a urinary tract infection (UTI) recently?
- Are you experiencing any bowel difficulties, such as constipation or accidents?
- Do you have any sexual or intimacy concerns?
- Are you experiencing any vision difficulties?
- How is your mobility?
- How often do you fall (or nearly fall) and why?
- How often do you exercise?
- Are you able to take your disease management agent as prescribed or are you having difficulty?
- How is your ability to perform self-care such as bathing, dressing, transfers, eating, meal preparation, and other chores?

Preparing for Annual Primary Care Evaluation

- Are you experiencing any difficulties with work?
- What type of social support do you have from family, friends, and your community?
- How much tobacco, alcohol, or other substances do you use?

Attention to these and other details can maximize your independence and quality of life (QOL). Taking the time to care for your primary and specialty needs is a great way to minimize difficulties you and your family may experience with MS and your health.[1]

---

[1] "Preparing for Your Multiple Sclerosis Office Visit," U.S. Department of Veterans Affairs (VA), February 13, 2024. Available online. URL: www.va.gov/MS/TREATING_MS/Whole_Health/Preparing_for_Your_MS_Office_Visit.asp. Accessed February 20, 2024.

Chapter 25 | Working with a Neurologist

NEUROLOGY'S ROLE IN MULTIPLE SCLEROSIS CARE
- Establish the correct diagnosis of multiple sclerosis (MS).
- Provide specialty care in outpatient MS clinic.
- Provide inpatient care for management of severe MS exacerbations.
- Perform lumbar punctures, if needed.
- Select disease modifying treatments and monitor their safety and effectiveness.
- Monitor the effects of MS with MRI.
- Partner with the U.S. Department of Veterans Affairs (VA) infusion clinic to provide IV medications or therapies.
- Partner with RCS-MS Clinic in managing functional impairments or MS related symptoms that affect quality of life (QOL).

REHABILITATION'S ROLE IN MS CARE
- Assess and manage medications for MS symptoms.
- Assess and manage MS symptoms such as fatigue, bowel and bladder problems, spasticity, pain, vision, and mood alteration.
- Assess and manage memory, swallowing, and speech problems.
- Assess and manage problems with mobility and doing a home exercise program.

- Assess and manage problems with self-care such as getting dressed, eating, getting on and off the toilet, and in and out of the shower.
- Assess for and prescribe equipment such as canes, walkers, wheelchairs, home safety equipment braces, and other adaptive technology.
- Assess and manage mood problems.
- Evaluate if there are VA or community resources that Veterans qualify for.
- Evaluate and make recommendations for leisure activities or help access community happenings despite disability.
- Vocational services.[1]

The clinical diagnosis of MS is made after thorough evaluation, usually by a neurologist or another provider with experience working with MS, and is not based on one specific physical finding, laboratory test, or symptom. Importantly, the diagnosis of MS relies on exclusion of other causes of symptoms and signs that might otherwise suggest MS but are accompanied by "red flags" that point to an alternative and unifying diagnosis. In addition, it is important to understand what imaging findings are and are not typical of MS to avoid misattributing magnetic resonance imaging (MRI) lesions to MS. The diagnosis of MS takes time and can be challenging.

The symptoms of MS can come and go, and they are not the same for every person. Since the diagnosis of MS is a clinical diagnosis, MRI and laboratory testing are not required. However, given the high sensitivity and specificity of MRI findings in MS, and the utility for monitoring disease and response to therapy, MRI is nearly universally conducted when possible.

An MRI has the ability to show dissemination in space with lesions in typical locations and dissemination in time with the presence of simultaneous enhancing and nonenhancing lesions or new lesion formation on a subsequent MRI. Consensus

---

[1] "Multiple Sclerosis (MS)," U.S. Department of Veterans Affairs (VA), March 15, 2024. Available online. URL: www.va.gov/puget-sound-health-care/programs/multiple-sclerosis-ms. Accessed April 26, 2024.

Working with a Neurologist

recommendations are to use brain MRI with and without contrast for initial diagnosis. Spinal cord imaging is indicated if the clinical exam localizes to the spinal cord, or the brain MRI does not demonstrate dissemination in space. The whole cord (cervical through lumbar) spinal cord imaging is advised with and without contrast; however, the bulk of the cord lesions occur in the cervical and thoracic cord.

Additional testing for the diagnosis of MS may be necessary, including blood tests and spinal fluid analysis. Elevated cerebrospinal fluid (CSF) oligoclonal bands, an elevated immunoglobulin G (IgG) index, and/or elevated synthetic rate are found in about 75 percent of people with MS. In patients with one clinical attack and evidence on two or more typical lesions on MRI, the presence of oligoclonal bands can establish dissemination in time (and thus a diagnosis of MS) with the 2017 McDonald Criteria. There is no one laboratory, MRI, or clinical test that definitively rules in or rules out MS.

Relapsing Multiple Sclerosis

Eighty-five percent of people with MS have a relapsing form of MS at onset. Relapsing MS diagnosis requires objective clinical evidence of two or more central nervous system (CNS) lesions (dissemination in space) that have occurred at different times (dissemination in time), or objective clinical evidence of one lesion with reasonable historical evidence of a prior attack. The reasonable historical evidence can be documented by a prior provider of symptoms and signs attributable to an acute CNS attack. A good patient historian can also give a description of symptoms that are typical for MS and thus can be the historical event. Descriptions of fully or partially reversible symptoms that describe optic neuritis, transverse myelitis (TM), brainstem syndrome, or other symptoms clearly referable to the CNS represent good historical evidence of a prior attack. Symptoms such as headache, poor cognition, fatigue, and generalized weakness, although they could be due to MS, are not specific for MS or even a CNS event and should not count as a historical attack. An MS attack should last at least 24 hours, usually lasts no more than one to two months and resolves fully or partly with residual symptoms. Dissemination of attacks in space and time is the cornerstone of MS diagnosis.

Primary Progressive Multiple Sclerosis

Fifteen percent of people with MS have a progressive form of disease at onset, defined as a gradual worsening of neurological symptoms and signs referable to the CNS for at least one year. Diagnosis of primary progressive MS can be more challenging and relies more heavily on ruling out other causes of symptoms. The MRI and spinal fluid evaluation is used more often in primary progressive MS to support the diagnosis. The 2017 McDonald Criteria also cover the requirements to diagnose primary progressive MS. It is important to distinguish relapsing from primary progressive MS as the treatments can be different.

Secondary Progressive Multiple Sclerosis

After approximately 15–20 years, about half of the people initially diagnosed with relapsing MS transition to secondary progressive MS. In this phase, there is a gradual worsening of neurological symptoms and signs between MS attacks. In many people, MS attacks eventually stop altogether, but some have both relapses and progression. It is important to recognize if a relapsing patient also has a progressive component between attacks to their disease as current MS therapies do not effectively slow the progressive aspect of MS. Secondary progressive MS does not have set criteria and is not part of any MS diagnostic criteria.

Clinically Isolated Syndrome

Clinically isolated syndrome (CIS) is a term that describes an isolated episode of neurological symptoms caused by inflammatory disease of the brain or spinal cord that do not meet 2017 McDonald criteria for MS. CIS can be monofocal, a single symptom such as vision loss from optic neuritis, or multifocal due to lesions in several locations.

Working with a Neurologist

In diagnosing CIS, the physician faces two challenges: first, to determine whether the person's symptoms are caused by CNS inflammation and not another process and second, to determine the likelihood that a person experiencing this type of demyelinating event is going to develop MS. A person with CIS has a higher risk (70–80%) of developing MS when the CIS is accompanied by MRI-detected brain lesions that are similar to those seen in MS (i.e., typical lesions). Conversely, there is a lower risk (20–30%) for MS when the MRI does not show brain lesions. A radiologist or neurologist trained in examining lesions is helpful in determining if lesions, if present, are typical of MS.

An accurate diagnosis of high- or low-risk CIS is important because people with a high-risk CIS are encouraged to begin treatment with a disease-modifying medication to delay or prevent a second neurologic episode and, therefore, the onset of MS. In addition, early treatment may minimize future disability caused by MS. Several medications are now approved by the U.S. Food and Drug Administration (FDA) for CIS.[2]

---

[2] "Diagnosing Multiple Sclerosis Using the McDonald Criteria," U.S. Department of Veterans Affairs (VA), July 6, 2022. Available online. URL: www.va.gov/MS/Professionals/diagnosis/Diagnosing_MS_Using_the_McDonald_Criteria.asp. Accessed February 22, 2024.

Chapter 26 | Diagnosing Multiple Sclerosis

Chapter Contents
Section 26.1—Imaging Tests and Procedures for Multiple
   Sclerosis 149
Section 26.2—Magnetic Resonance Imaging 151
Section 26.3—Kurtzke Expanded Disability Status Scale 154

Section 26.1 | Imaging Tests and Procedures for Multiple Sclerosis

Diagnostic tests and procedures are vital tools that help physicians confirm or rule out a neurological disorder or other medical condition. A century ago, the only way to make a definite diagnosis for many neurological disorders was to perform an autopsy after someone had died. Today, new instruments and techniques allow scientists to assess the living brain and monitor nervous system activity as it occurs. Doctors now have powerful and accurate tools to better diagnose disease and to test how well a particular therapy may be working. The following procedures are used to diagnose multiple sclerosis (MS).

LUMBAR PUNCTURE

The lumbar puncture may be done as an inpatient or as an outpatient procedure. During the lumbar puncture, the person will either lie on one side, with knees close to the chest, or lean forward while sitting on a table, bed, or massage chair. The person's back will be cleaned and injected with a local anesthetic. The injection may cause a slight stinging sensation. Once the anesthetic has taken effect, a special needle is inserted between the vertebrae into the spinal sac, and a small amount of fluid (usually about three teaspoons) is withdrawn for testing. Most people will only feel a sensation of pressure as the needle is inserted. Generally, people are asked to lie flat for an hour or two to reduce the after-effect of headache. There is a small risk of nerve root injury or infection from a lumbar puncture. The procedure takes about 45 minutes.

EVOKED POTENTIALS

Evoked potentials, also called "evoked response," measure the electrical signals to the brain generated by hearing, touch, or sight. Evoked potentials are used to test sight and hearing (especially in infants and young children) and can help diagnose neurological conditions such as MS, spinal cord injury, and acoustic neuroma (small tumors of the acoustic nerve). Evoked potentials are also used to monitor brain activity among coma patients and confirm brain death.

Testing may take place in a doctor's office or hospital setting. One set of electrodes is attached to the person's scalp with conducting paste. The electrodes measure the brain's electrical response to stimuli. A machine records the amount of time it takes for impulses generated by stimuli to reach the brain.

- **Auditory evoked potentials (also called "brain stem auditory evoked response")**. These can assess hearing loss and damage to the acoustic nerve and auditory pathways in the brain stem. The person being tested sits in a soundproof room and wears headphones. Clicking sounds are delivered one at a time to one ear while a masking sound is sent to the other ear. Each ear is usually tested twice, and the entire procedure takes about 45 minutes.
- **Visual evoked potentials.** These potentials detect loss of vision from optic nerve damage (e.g., from MS). The person sits close to a screen and is asked to focus in the center of a shifting checkerboard pattern. One eye is tested at a time. Each eye is usually tested twice. Testing takes 30–45 minutes.
- **Somatosensory evoked potentials (SSEPs).** SSEPs measure responses from electrical stimuli to the nerves. In addition to electrodes on the scalp, electrodes are pasted to the arms, leg, and back to measure the signal as it travels from the peripheral nerves to the brain. Tiny electrical shocks are delivered by electrodes pasted to the skin over a nerve in an arm or leg. SSEPs may be used to help diagnose MS, spinal cord compression or injury, and certain metabolic or degenerative diseases. SSEP tests usually take longer than an hour.[1]

---

[1] "Neurological Diagnostic Tests and Procedures," National Institute of Neurological Disorders and Stroke (NINDS), April 2019. Available online. URL: https://catalog.ninds.nih.gov/sites/default/files/publications/neurological-diagnostic-tests-procedures.pdf. Accessed February 22, 2024.

Section 26.2 | Magnetic Resonance Imaging

Magnetic resonance imaging (MRI) is an excellent resource for people with multiple sclerosis (MS). MRI studies provide a safe and noninvasive way to obtain detailed images of the brain and spinal cord, without any radiation exposure.

As patient access to medical records continues to increase, patients can sometimes see the images or read the MRI report even before discussing them with their neurologist. This presents a challenge since the language in the report and the importance of certain findings are not always easily understood by someone who is not trained to read them. It is best to review an MRI report with your physician, whether face-to-face or by telephone or webcam, to make sure that the radiology report is translated with your specific health and diagnosis in mind.

MAGNETIC RESONANCE IMAGING BREAKDOWN

An MRI is made by combining multiple images, with each image being an extremely thin slice of the brain or spinal cord. Some MRIs progress in the direction of the feet to the top of the head, which means on the computer screen, the right side of the image is the left side of the body. Every MRI can be rearranged by computer to show different perspectives, providing even more information about potentially damaged brain tissue caused by MS.

Each MRI can also be taken in different formats, also known as "sequences," such as a filter in photography. Each sequence has its own advantages and disadvantages. T1 sequences show detailed anatomy of the brain and spinal cord, which is helpful in identifying "black holes," which represent areas of atrophy or shrinking of previously injured brain tissue. These black holes can also be called "hypointense" on the MRI report. T2 MRI sequences are used to highlight areas of demyelination, which happens when the outer layer of the neurons is damaged due to MS activity. T2 sequences can be used to count the total number of MS lesions, which look like bright white spots on T2 sequences, and can be called "hyperintense." To help identify new or active areas of disease, a special contrast dye can be given by intravenous (IV) during the MRI. This makes it easier to compare new MS activity, older injury, and healthy brain tissue. The contrast dye contains a metal called "gadolinium," made nontoxic for medical use.

Altogether, T1 sequences show any old areas of atrophy or black holes, T2 sequences help show the overall number of MS lesions in the brain or spinal cord (also known as "MS lesion burden"), and contrast-enhanced sequences show any new and active MS lesions (also known as "enhancing lesions").

MAGNETIC RESONANCE IMAGING "IMPRESSIONS"

Every MRI has a radiologist review the entire study very carefully, looking for both normal brain tissue and potential signs of disease. Sometimes an MRI reviewed by a radiologist can provide enough evidence to make a diagnosis. But in the case of MS, it takes a combination of the MRI with the patient's clinical symptoms, history, and neurological examination to make the diagnosis. MS diagnosis involves meeting several clinical and imaging criteria, in addition to making sure no other disease can explain the patient's presentation. In other words, the patient's neurologist needs to look for signs of MS while making sure nothing else could explain the patient's current condition at the same time.

While it is true that almost all people with MS will have evidence of brain lesions on MRI, not all people with brain lesions have MS. Therefore, an MRI report lists many possibilities that could explain the MRI's particular appearance. This list of possibilities always requires thoughtful review by the patient's health-care provider and must always consider the broader picture.

An MRI alone cannot be used to see how well a patient is doing; it must always be studied with the patient in mind. An MRI cannot take the place of regular follow-up visits, clear communication of symptoms, and neurological examination by a patient's health-care provider.

One of the most valuable aspects of an MRI is comparison of studies over time, to see how they change. To improve the accuracy of MRI comparison, it is best to get the studies completed at the same location. This makes it more likely that the techniques to capture and read the MRI are the same between studies. If you cannot get your MRI study completed at the same place you had it done last time, ask for a copy of the MRI (both the imaging files and the report) from the last place, both for your own records and to share with your providers.

While it is always better to review an MRI report with your health-care provider, with a little bit of understanding of terminology, it is possible to make some sense of your MRI report even before communicating with your doctor.[2]

DIAGNOSING MULTIPLE SCLEROSIS USING THE MCDONALD CRITERIA

The diagnosis of MS is by clinical criteria with support as necessary from MRI and spinal fluid analysis. The criteria have evolved over time to allow more rapid diagnosis of MS and thus permit earlier treatment of MS. The diagnosis of MS can be challenging and is focused on excluding MS mimics that have alternative treatments. Given that MS is a clinical diagnosis that can evolve over time, careful follow-up of patients is necessary to confirm that MS, once diagnosed, remains the best possible diagnosis.

Diagnostic Criteria

Diagnostic criteria have evolved over time from the Schumacher Criteria (1965), to the Poser Criteria (1983), and finally to the McDonald Criteria (2001). The McDonald Criteria were developed by an international panel in association with the National MS Society of America, modified in 2005, and revised again in 2010 and 2017. The McDonald Criteria revisions enable more rapid diagnosis of MS and thus permit earlier treatment of MS. For clinical research trials, the McDonald Criteria (www.va.gov/MS/Professionals/diagnosis/Updated_McDonald_Criteria_2017.pdf) ensure that those without a definite diagnosis of MS are not enrolled.

---

[2] "Understanding Your MRI Report," U.S. Department of Veterans Affairs (VA), February 8, 2023. Available online. URL: www.va.gov/MS/Veterans/about_MS/Understanding_Your_MRI_Report.asp. Accessed February 22, 2024.

Abnormal Brain Magnetic Resonance Imaging

Occasionally, people get brain MRIs for reasons other than suspected MS such as a car accident or migraines. Sometimes these MRIs look similar to ones from people with MS. MRI mimics of MS are numerous, and not all radiologists are familiar with current MRI criteria. It is important to remember that the radiologist cannot make the diagnosis of MS as it is a clinical diagnosis based on history and neurological examination. Patients with abnormal MRIs that are suspicious of MS should be evaluated for a history of events typical of MS or neurological findings referable to the central nervous system (CNS). Usually, a neurologist is best able to perform this evaluation.

Patients diagnosed prior to MRIs or by another provider deserve to have the original and ongoing basis for their diagnosis reviewed in light of the 2017 McDonald Criteria. This is important as MS treatment comes with risks to the patient, which can be avoided with correct diagnosis.[3]

Section 26.3 | Kurtzke Expanded Disability Status Scale

The Kurtzke Disability Status Scale (DSS) was developed by Dr. John Kurtzke in the 1950s to measure the disability status of people with multiple sclerosis (MS). The purpose was to create an objective approach to quantify the level of functioning that could be widely used by health-care providers diagnosing MS. The scale was modified several times to more accurately reflect the levels of disabilities clinically observed. The scale was renamed the Kurtzke Expanded Disability Status Scale (EDSS).

The EDSS provides a total score on a scale that ranges from 0 to 10 (see Table 26.1). The first levels 1.0 to 4.5 refer to people with a

---

[3] "Diagnosing Multiple Sclerosis Using the McDonald Criteria," U.S. Department of Veterans Affairs (VA), July 6, 2022. Available online. URL: www.va.gov/MS/Professionals/diagnosis/Diagnosing_MS_Using_the_McDonald_Criteria.asp. Accessed February 22, 2024.

Diagnosing Multiple Sclerosis

high degree of ambulatory ability and the subsequent levels 5.0 to 9.5 refer to the loss of ambulatory ability.

Table 26.1. Kurtzke Expanded Disability Status Scale (EDSS)

0	Normal neurological exam (all grade 0 in all Functional System (FS) scores*).
1	No disability, minimal signs in one FS* (i.e., grade 1).
1.5	No disability, minimal signs in more than one FS* (more than 1 FS grade 1).
2	Minimal disability in one FS (one FS grade 2, others 0 or 1).
2.5	Minimal disability in two FS (two FS grade 2, others 0 or 1).
3	Moderate disability in one FS (one FS grade 3, others 0 or 1) or mild disability in three or four FS (three or four FS grade 2, others 0 or 1) though fully ambulatory.
3.5	Fully ambulatory but with moderate disability in one FS (one grade 3) and one or two FS grade 2; or two FS grade 3 (others 0 or 1) or five grade 2 (others 0 or 1).
4	Fully ambulatory without aid, self-sufficient, up, and about some 12 hours a day despite relatively severe disability consisting of one FS grade 4 (others 0 or 1), or combination of lesser grades exceeding limits of previous steps; able to walk without aid or rest greater than 500 meters.
4.5	Fully ambulatory without aid, up and about much of the day, able to work a full day, may otherwise have some limitation of full activity or require minimal assistance; characterized by relatively severe disability usually consisting of one FS grade 4 (others or 1) or combinations of lesser grades exceeding limits of previous steps; able to walk without aid or rest greater than 300 meters.
5	Ambulatory without aid or rest for about 200 meters; disability severe enough to impair full daily activities (e.g., to work a full day without special provisions; usual FS equivalents are one grade 5 alone, others 0 or 1; or combinations of lesser grades usually exceeding specifications for step 4.0).
5.5	Ambulatory without aid for about 100 meters; disability severe enough to preclude full daily activities; (Usual FS equivalents are one grade 5 alone, others 0 or 1; or combination of lesser grades usually exceeding those for step 4.0).
6	Intermittent or unilateral constant assistance (cane, crutch, and brace) required to walk about 100 meters with or without resting; (Usual FS equivalents are combinations with more than two FS grade 3+).
6.5	Constant bilateral assistance (canes, crutches, and braces) required to walk about 20 meters without resting; (Usual FS equivalents are combinations with more than two FS grade 3+).

Table 26.1. Continued

7	Unable to walk beyond approximately 5 meters even with aid, essentially restricted to wheelchair; wheels self in standard wheelchair and transfers alone; up and about in wheelchair some 12 hours a day; (Usual FS equivalents are combinations with more than one FS grade 4+; very rarely pyramidal grade 5 alone).
7.5	Unable to take more than a few steps; restricted to wheelchair; may need aid in transfer; wheels self but cannot carry on in standard wheelchair a full day; may require a motorized wheelchair; (Usual FS equivalents are combinations with more than one FS grade 4+).
8	Essentially restricted to bed or chair or perambulated in a wheelchair but may be out of bed itself much of the day; retains many self-care functions; generally has effective use of arms; (Usual FS equivalents are combinations, generally grade 4+ in several systems).
8.5	Essentially restricted to bed much of day; has some effective use of arm(s); retains some self-care functions; (Usual FS equivalents are combinations, generally 4+ in several systems).
9	Helpless bed patient; can communicate and eat; (Usual FS equivalents are combinations, mostly grade 4+).
9.5	Totally helpless bed patient; unable to communicate effectively or eat/swallow; (Usual FS equivalents are combinations, almost all grade 4+).
10	Death due to MS

* Excludes cerebral function grade 1.
Note 1: EDSS steps 1.0 to 4.5 refer to patients who are fully ambulatory, and the precise step number is defined by the Functional System score(s). EDSS steps 5.0 to 9.5 are defined by the impairment to ambulation and usual equivalents in Functional Systems scores are provided.
Note 2: EDSS should not change by 1.0 step unless there is a change in the same direction of at least one step in at least one FS.

In addition, it also provides eight subscale measurements called "Functional System" (FS) scores. The levels of function within each category refer to the eight functional systems affected by MS.

Eight Functional Systems and Their Abbreviations
- Pyramidal (P; motor function)
- Cerebellar (C11)
- Brainstem (BS)
- Sensory (S)
- Bowel and Bladder (BB)

Diagnosing Multiple Sclerosis

- Visual (V)
- Cerebral or Mental (Cb)
- Other (O)

The FS scores are scored on a scale of 0 (low level of problems) to 5 or 6 (high level of problems) to best reflect the level of disability observed clinically. The "Other" category consists of any other neurologic findings attributed to MS and is dichotomous, with 0 as none and 1 as any present.

In contrast, the total EDSS score is determined by two factors: gait and FS scores. EDSS scores below 4.0 are determined by the FS scores alone. People with EDSS scores of 4.0 and above may have some degree of gait impairment. Scores between 4.0 and 9.5 are determined by both gait abilities and the FS scores. For simplicity, many experts gauge the EDSS scores between 4.0 and 9.5 entirely by gait, without considering the FS scores. The EDSS is widely used and accepted as a valid tool to clinically measure and evaluate the level of functioning of MS patients.[4]

---

[4] "Kurtzke Expanded Disability Status Scale," U.S. Department of Veterans Affairs (VA), March 18, 2021. Available online. URL: www.va.gov/MS/Professionals/diagnosis/Kurtzke_Expanded_Disability_Status_Scale.asp. Accessed February 22, 2024.

Chapter 27 | Treatment Options for Multiple Sclerosis

There is no cure for multiple sclerosis (MS), but there are treatments that can reduce the number and severity of relapses and delay the long-term disability progression of the disease.

TREATMENTS FOR ATTACKS
- **Corticosteroids**. Intravenous (infused into a vein) methylprednisolone is prescribed over the course of three to five days. Intravenous steroids quickly and potently suppress the immune system and reduce inflammation. They may be followed by a tapered dose of oral corticosteroids. Clinical trials have shown that these drugs hasten recovery from MS attacks but do not alter the long-term outcome of the disease.
- **Plasma exchange (plasmapheresis)**. It can treat severe flare-ups in people with relapsing forms of MS who do not have a good response to methylprednisolone. Plasma exchange involves taking blood out of the body and removing components in the blood's plasma that are thought to be harmful. The rest of the blood, plus replacement plasma, is then transfused back into the body. This treatment has not been shown to be effective for secondary progressive or chronic progressive MS.

DISEASE-MODIFYING TREATMENTS

Current therapies approved by the U.S. Food and Drug Administration (FDA) for MS are designed to modulate or suppress the inflammatory reactions of the disease. They are most effective for relapsing-remitting MS at early stages of the disease.

Injectable medications include the following:
- **Beta interferon drugs**. The most common medications to treat MS. Interferons are signaling molecules that regulate immune cells. Potential side effects of these drugs include flu-like symptoms (which usually fade with continued therapy), depression, or elevation of liver enzymes. Some individuals will notice a decrease in the effectiveness of the drugs after 18–24 months of treatment. If flare-ups occur or symptoms worsen, doctors may switch treatment to alternative drugs.
- **Glatiramer acetate**. Changes the balance of immune cells in the body but how it works is not entirely clear. Side effects are usually mild and consist of local injection site reactions or swelling.

Infusion treatments include the following:
- **Natalizumab**. It is administered intravenously once a month. It works by preventing cells of the immune system from entering the brain and spinal cord. It is very effective but is associated with an increased risk of a serious and potentially fatal viral infection of the brain called "progressive multifocal leukoencephalopathy" (PML). Natalizumab is generally recommended only for individuals who have not responded well to or who are unable to tolerate other first-line therapies.
- **Ocrelizumab**. It is administered intravenously every six months and treats adults with relapsing or primary progressive forms of MS. It is the only FDA-approved disease-modifying therapy for primary-progressive MS. The drug targets the circulating immune cells that produce antibodies, which also play a role in the

formation of MS lesions. Side effects include infusion-related reactions and increased risk of infections. Ocrelizumab may increase the risk of cancer as well.
- **Alemtuzumab.** It is administered for five consecutive days, followed by three days of infusions one year later. It targets proteins on the surface of immune cells. Because this drug increases the risk of autoimmune disorders, it is recommended for those who have had inadequate responses to two or more MS therapies.
- **Mitoxantrone.** It is administered intravenously four times a year, has been approved for especially severe forms of relapsing-remitting and secondary-progressive MS. Side effects include the development of certain types of blood cancers in up to 1 percent of those with MS, as well as with heart damage. This drug should be considered as a last resort to treat people with a form of MS that leads to rapid loss of function and for whom other treatments did not work.

Oral treatments include the following:
- **Fingolimod.** It is a once-daily medication that reduces the MS relapse rate in adults and children. It is the first FDA-approved drug to treat MS in adolescents and children aged 10 years and older. The drug prevents white blood cells (WBCs) called "lymphocytes" from leaving the lymph nodes and entering the blood, brain, and spinal cord. Fingolimod may result in a slow heart rate and eye problems when first taken. Fingolimod can also increase the risk of infections, such as herpes virus infections, or in rare cases be associated with PML.
- **Dimethyl fumarate.** It is a twice-daily medication used to treat relapsing forms of MS. Its exact mechanism of action is not currently known. Side effects of dimethyl fumarate are flushing, diarrhea, nausea, and lowered WBC count.
- **Teriflunomide.** It is a once-daily medication that reduces the rate of proliferation of activated immune

cells. Teriflunomide side effects can include nausea, diarrhea, liver damage, and hair loss.
- **Cladribine.** It is administered as two courses of tablets about one year apart. Cladribine targets certain types of WBC that drive immune attacks in MS. The drug may increase the risk of developing cancer and should be considered for individuals who have not responded well to other MS treatments.
- **Diroximel fumarate.** It is a twice-daily drug similar to dimethyl fumarate (brand name Tecfidera) but with fewer gastrointestinal side effects. Scientists suspect these drugs, which have been approved to treat secondary-progressive MS, reduce damage to the brain and spinal cord by making the immune response less inflammatory, although their exact mechanism of action is poorly understood.
- **Siponimod tablets (Mayzent).** It is taken orally and has a similar mechanism of action to fingolimod. Siponimod has been approved by the FDA to treat secondary-progressive MS.

Clinical trials have shown that cladribine, diroximel fumarate, and dimethyl fumarate decrease the number of relapses, delay the progress of physical disability, and slow the development of brain lesions.

MANAGING MULTIPLE SCLEROSIS SYMPTOMS

Multiple sclerosis causes a variety of symptoms that can interfere with daily activities but can usually be treated or managed. Many of these issues are best treated by neurologists who have advanced training in the treatment of MS and who can prescribe specific medications to treat these problems.
- **Eye and vision problems.** These are common in people with MS but rarely result in permanent blindness. Inflammation of the optic nerve (optic neuritis) or damage to the myelin that covers the nerve fibers in the visual system can cause blurred or grayed vision,

temporary blindness in one eye, loss of normal color vision, depth perception, or loss of vision in parts of the visual field. Uncontrolled horizontal or vertical eye movements (nystagmus), "jumping vision" (opsoclonus), and double vision (diplopia) are common in people with MS. Intravenous steroid medications, special eyeglasses, and periodically resting the eyes may be helpful.
- **Muscle weakness and spasticity.** It is common in MS. Mild spasticity can be managed by stretching and exercising muscles using water therapy, yoga, or physical therapy. Medications such as gabapentin or baclofen can reduce spasticity. It is very important that people with MS stay physically active because physical inactivity can contribute to worsening stiffness, weakness, pain, fatigue, and other symptoms.
- **Tremor.** Uncontrollable shaking (tremor) develops in some people with MS. Assistive devices and weights attached to utensils or even limbs are sometimes helpful for people with tremor. Deep brain stimulation (DBS) and drugs, such as clonazepam, may also be useful.
- **Problems with walking and balance.** It occurs in many people with MS. The most common walking problem is ataxia—unsteady, uncoordinated movements—due to damage to the areas of the brain that coordinate muscle balance. People with severe ataxia generally benefit from the use of a cane, walker, or other assistive device. Physical therapy can also reduce walking problems. The FDA has approved the drug dalfampridine to improve walking speed in people with MS.
- **Fatigue.** It is a common symptom of MS and may be both physical (e.g., tiredness in the arms or legs) and cognitive (slowed processing speed or mental exhaustion). Daily physical activity programs of mild-to-moderate intensity can significantly reduce fatigue, although people should avoid excessive physical activity and minimize exposure to hot weather conditions or

ambient temperature. Other drugs that may reduce fatigue include amantadine, methylphenidate, and modafinil. Occupational therapy can help people learn how to walk using an assistive device or in a way that saves physical energy. Stress management programs, relaxation training, membership in an MS support group, or individual psychotherapy may help some people.
- **Pain from MS.** It can be felt in different parts of the body. Trigeminal neuralgia (facial pain) is treated with anticonvulsant or antispasmodic drugs or less commonly painkillers. Central pain, a syndrome caused by damage to the brain and/or spinal cord, can be treated with gabapentin and nortriptyline. Treatments for chronic back or other musculoskeletal pain may include heat, massage, ultrasound, and physical therapy.
- **Problems with bladder control and constipation.** It may include urinary frequency, urgency, or the loss of bladder control. A small number of individuals retain large amounts of urine. Medical treatments are available for bladder-related problems. Constipation is also common and can be treated with a high-fiber diet, laxatives, and stool softeners.
- **Sexual dysfunction.** It can result from damage to nerves running through the spinal cord. Sexual problems may also stem from MS symptoms such as fatigue, cramped or spastic muscles, and psychological factors. Some of these problems can be corrected with medications. Psychological counseling may also be helpful.
- **Clinical depression.** It is frequent among people with MS. MS may cause depression as part of the disease process and chemical imbalance in the brain. Depression can intensify symptoms of fatigue, pain, and sexual dysfunction. It is most often treated with cognitive behavioral therapy (CBT), and selective

serotonin reuptake inhibitor (SSRI) antidepressant medications, which are less likely than other antidepressant medications to cause fatigue.
- **Inappropriate and involuntary expressions of laughter, crying, or anger.** Symptoms of a condition called "pseudobulbar affect"—sometimes are associated with MS. These expressions are often incongruent with mood; for example, people with MS may cry when they are actually happy or laugh when they are not especially happy. The combination treatment of the drugs dextromethorphan and quinidine can treat pseudobulbar affect, as can other drugs such as amitriptyline or citalopram.
- **Cognitive impairment.** A decline in the ability to think quickly and clearly and to remember easily affects up to three-quarters of people with MS. These cognitive changes may appear at the same time as the physical symptoms, or they may develop gradually over time. Drugs such as donepezil may be helpful in some cases.[1]

MANAGING SPASTICITY WITH AN INTRATHECAL BACLOFEN PUMP

People living with MS can experience muscle stiffness, pain, jerking, weakness, or difficulty coordinating their movements. This is called "spasticity." Spasticity is a disorder of the muscles and nerves commonly seen in people living with MS. Due to MS plaques in the brain and spinal cord, the body's normal ability to control muscle contractions and muscle relaxation is lost. Spasticity can be constant or come and go. Spasticity can be triggered by moving the limbs or irritation such as a wound or urinary tract infection. When spasticity is severe, it can limit a person's ability to walk, get dressed, complete personal hygiene, sit comfortably, or can cause pain.

---

[1] "Multiple Sclerosis: Hope through Research," National Institute of Neurological Disorders and Stroke (NINDS), August 2020. Available online. URL: https://catalog.ninds.nih.gov/sites/default/files/publications/multiple-sclerosis-hope-through-research_0.pdf. Accessed February 22, 2024.

How Is Spasticity Treated?

There are many ways to treat spasticity and frequently multiple treatments are used at the same time. Daily stretching and strengthening are usually tried first for mild spasticity. Medications, such as baclofen, tizanidine, gabapentin, clonidine, dantrolene, or in some instances, diazepam can be used. Botulinum toxin injections can be used when spasticity only affects a limited area, such as one leg or arm. Bracing and surgery can also be used in certain cases. Delivering liquid baclofen into the spinal canal, called "intrathecal baclofen" (ITB), can also be used if other treatments are unsuccessful.

What Is Intrathecal Baclofen Therapy?

Intrathecal baclofen therapy is when liquid baclofen is delivered around the spinal cord. A small, round pump is surgically placed under the skin in the abdomen. A thin tube (catheter) attaches to the pump and goes around the abdomen to the back and is inserted into the spinal canal. Usually, you will be able to see and feel the pump. You will not be able to see or feel the catheter. The pump generally holds enough medication to last several months and is refilled in an office visit. The battery for the pump will last around seven years.

What Are the Benefits of Intrathecal Baclofen?

Medications used to treat spasticity can have side effects, including dizziness, fatigue, or sleepiness. With ITB, since it is going directly to the spinal cord, it uses up to 100 times less medication to get the same effect. Additionally, the medication goes right to the spinal cord and may be more effective.

Who Is the Best Candidate for Intrathecal Baclofen Therapy?

The best candidates for ITB are people whose spasticity or spasms are not well controlled with other treatment options. They will need to be able to come in regularly for management of the pump. ITB therapy can be appropriate for people living with MS and should be considered if people are able to walk or are restricted to their bed. The goals of ITB therapy could include improving or maintaining the ability to walk, decreasing painful spasms, maintaining joint mobility, protecting the skin, doing personal hygiene activities, or making it easier to sit in a chair.

What Is an Intrathecal Baclofen Screening Test?

Prior to getting a pump, most physicians will perform a screening test or refer you to a physician who does these tests. For the screening test, a dose of baclofen is injected into the spinal canal through a lumbar puncture, also called a "spinal tap." You may have had this when you were diagnosed with MS. The test dose will give you and your doctor an idea if this medication is effective. This screening test may take place in a clinic or during a hospital admission.

During a positive response, the legs may become temporarily weak. This goes away usually in four to eight hours. During this time, you will be monitored by your doctor or physical therapist. They will monitor your blood pressure and heart rate, improvement in your symptoms, and note any negative side effects you may have. When the results of the medication fade, you will be sent home. Usually this is the same day. Rarely, you may have to spend the night in the hospital. The effects of the ITB therapy are not permanent. Although most doctors do a test dose to see if you are responsive to ITB, the test dose does not always predict exactly what it will be like with an ITB pump.

How Is the Pump Implanted?

After the test dose, you and your doctor will decide if putting an ITB pump in surgically is right for you. The surgery will be scheduled for another admission and will be done by a surgeon who is familiar with this procedure. Most people are sent home the following day after the pump is implanted. Rarely, you may need to stay in the hospital for a couple of days while the dose is adjusted, and you receive physical or occupational therapy.

What Is Done to Manage the Intrathecal Baclofen Pump after Implantation?

After the pump is implanted, the dose will be noninvasively adjusted in your doctor's office. Initially, this may be weekly to increase the pump dose and wean off oral spasticity medications. A stable dose is usually reached in several months. The daily dose can continue to be changed as needed. Depending on how much baclofen you use, your pump will need to be refilled every month to every six months. The pump has an alarm that will alert you if the pump runs out of medication or the battery is no longer functioning. Another surgery will be needed to replace the pump when the battery dies, or if there is a problem with the pump or catheter malfunctioning.

Severe consequences are rare, but there is a chance of life-threatening events such as getting too much baclofen (an overdose) or too little baclofen (withdrawal). Warning signs of an overdose can include drowsiness, lightheadedness, dizziness, difficulty breathing, seizures, lower than normal body temperature, or loss of consciousness. Warning signs of withdrawal can include increase or return of spasticity, itching, low blood pressure, lightheadedness, or a tingling sensation. If you have these symptoms, you will need to seek immediate care such as seeing your doctor or going to the emergency room.[2]

ROLE OF EXERCISE AND MOVEMENT

Exercise is a well-established pillar of a healthy lifestyle. It has the ability to prevent and treat a wide range of illnesses from cardiovascular disease to depression and from dementia to osteoarthritis. However, until recently, physicians often recommended that MS patients avoid exercise. The main concerns included exercise causing a rise in the body temperature that might trigger symptoms in heat-sensitive patients and exacerbate MS-related fatigue. The Uhthoff phenomenon describes a transient amblyopia that can occur with exercise or overheating. Fortunately, these symptoms

---

[2] "Managing Spasticity with an Intrathecal Baclofen Pump," U.S. Department of Veterans Affairs (VA), February 13, 2024. Available online. URL: www.va.gov/MS/Veterans/symptoms_of_MS/Managing_Spasticity_with_an_Intrathecal_Baclofen_Pump.asp. Accessed February 22, 2024.

Treatment Options for Multiple Sclerosis

are reversible and are not thought to be triggers of exacerbations. Also reassuring is that normal exercise does not significantly raise the core temperature.

Implementing an exercise program requires an initial assessment of a person's current functional status and limitations. Patients with significant mobility needs, weakness, or spasticity should create an exercise plan with the help of a physical therapist or other person with experience in this area. For those with significant impairments, exercise programs can start with passive range-of-motion exercises, then advance to flexibility and active range-of-motion exercises. If that is well tolerated, more integrated exercises such as walking, swimming, or yoga can be initiated. If the goal is improved mobility, weight-bearing exercises should be included. Water-based exercises can be a good substitute for some patients. For those with few or no mobility issues, recommendations mirror those without MS: Find an activity you like to do, start slowly, and stick with it! Refer to Moving the Body (www.va.gov/WHOLEHEALTHLIBRARY/overviews/moving-the-body.asp) for additional information.[3]

---

[3] "Multiple Sclerosis," U.S. Department of Veterans Affairs (VA), February 9, 2022. Available online. URL: www.va.gov/WHOLEHEALTHLIBRARY/tools/multiple-sclerosis.asp. Accessed April 24, 2024.

Chapter 28 | Plasmapheresis

WHAT IS PLASMAPHERESIS?
Autoimmune diseases are usually treated with medicines that calm down the immune system or lessen swelling in the body tissues. However, using these drugs for a long time or in large doses can harm the body. To avoid relying solely on medication, scientists have developed an approach called "plasmapheresis." This process is similar to dialysis and is also known as "plasma exchange," where the liquid part, the plasma, is separated from the blood and discarded. The blood components are then returned to the body, along with the plasma substitute. This procedure successfully treats some autoimmune diseases, such as multiple sclerosis (MS), Guillain-Barré syndrome (GBS), Miller-Fisher syndrome (MFS), chronic inflammatory demyelinating polyneuropathy (CIDP), Goodpasture syndrome, and Lambert-Eaton syndrome.

The immune system produces antibodies to protect the body from infections such as bacteria, viruses, and other invaders. However, when the antibodies fail to recognize self and nonself, they become autoantibodies and attack their own cells, tissues, or organs. Plasma exchange is a process that can help remove autoantibodies from the blood.

REQUIREMENTS FOR PLASMA DONORS
To make sure donors and patients are safe, there are some requirements donors must meet. Generally, donors should:
- be at least 18 years old
- weigh at least 110 pounds
- be in good health

When you give plasma for the first time, you will complete an extensive medical history screening and a doctor will give you a physical exam. During the exam, and before all future plasma donations, you will also have to test negative for certain viruses, including hepatitis and human immunodeficiency virus (HIV).[1]

Plasma can only be used after you give two times. You must return to the same plasma center within six months and give again before any of your plasma can be used. This is another safety precaution. Plasma collection in the United States is regulated by the U.S. Food and Drug Administration (FDA), which requires two separate tests on a person's plasma to make sure it is safe to share with others.

Plasma regenerates quickly. With proper hydration, your blood volume returns to normal within 48 hours. Because of this, you can give plasma twice in any 7-day period, but no more than once in a 48-hour period.

You can typically schedule a return visit while you are at the plasma center. Many people choose to set up a series of visits. Repeat, committed visits are the best way to support our growing need for plasma.[2]

PROCEDURE FOR PLASMAPHERESIS

Anesthesia is generally not necessary for the plasmapheresis treatment itself, but local anesthesia may be used for the insertion of two relatively large needles. Once the needles are positioned, patients may feel discomfort but not pain for the rest of the procedure.

Before plasmapheresis, the patient is positioned in a reclining chair or asked to lie down. Two tubes (catheters or needles) are inserted, one in a large vein in the arm and the other in the opposite arm, foot, groin area, or shoulder. Blood is removed through one of the tubes and passed into an apheresis machine or cell separator. This device separates the plasma from the blood cells

---

[1] "Find Out If You Can Give Plasma," U.S. Department of Health and Human Services (HHS), September 27, 2022. Available online. URL: www.hhs.gov/givingequalsliving/giveplasma/can-i-give. Accessed April 30, 2024.

[2] "The Process for Giving Plasma, Step-by-Step," U.S. Department of Health and Human Services (HHS), September 27, 2022. Available online. URL: www.hhs.gov/givingequalsliving/giveplasma/giving-process. Accessed April 30, 2024.

Plasmapheresis

by spinning at high speed or passing the blood through a membrane with tiny pores, allowing only the plasma to pass through.

The extracted plasma containing the autoantibodies is then discarded. The substitute (replacement) plasma is combined with blood cells and reintroduced into the body through the other tube. The amount of blood outside the body at any given time during the procedure is generally less than the amount a donor would contribute at a blood bank.

Plasmapheresis is usually an outpatient procedure which takes one to three hours. For an average patient, treatments are repeated 6–10 times over the span of 2–10 weeks. The length and number of treatments depend on the diagnosis and the patient's general condition.

BEFORE THE PROCEDURE

Before plasmapheresis, the patient is examined by their physician. The health-care provider collects a complete medical history and reviews all medications to decide if the patient needs to stop certain medications before and after treatment.

To make the procedure go smoothly, practice the following:
- Getting a good sleep the night before the procedure is essential.
- Stay hydrated by drinking fluids in the days leading to the procedure.
- It is recommended to wear loose-fitting clothes that allow rolling the sleeves above the elbows.
- Bring a book to read or a portable music device with headphones to help pass the time.

POST-PROCEDURE

After plasmapheresis, the patient can leave the hospital or medical center after resting briefly. Since many people feel tired or weak after plasmapheresis, the patient will need someone to drive them home. Care must be taken to follow the doctor's instructions regarding medication dosages and to prevent infection. The patient may show improvement within days or, at most, a few weeks, and the treatment's positive effects last several months. However, since plasmapheresis is a temporary treatment, the procedure may have to be repeated on a regular basis.

RISKS AND COMPLICATIONS OF PLASMAPHERESIS

Although plasmapheresis is a safe therapeutic procedure, and complications do not occur often, like most medical procedures, it does carry some risks. Awareness of these risks may help the patient to be better prepared. A health-care provider should be contacted immediately if any serious complications develop.

A few of the possible risks and complications include:
- bleeding caused by the medication given to prevent clotting during the procedure
- severe bleeding may lead to irregular heartbeats or seizures
- low blood pressure
- dizziness, blurred vision, sweating, and abdominal cramps
- swelling, bruises, or rashes where needles or tubes were inserted
- fatigue, weakness, or joint pain
- infection
- anaphylaxis, a potentially dangerous reaction to the solutions used in plasma replacement (The procedure must be stopped if this complication occurs.)
- excessive suppression of the immune system during plasma exchange (This generally resolves in a short time as the body produces more antibodies.)

Plasmapheresis is not a disease-modifying therapy for chronic cases of MS as it cannot reverse the damage that has already occurred. The procedure is commonly used to alleviate symptoms and provide rapid relief for MS patients experiencing acute relapses that do not respond to steroids.

References
"Facts about Plasmapheresis," Muscular Dystrophy Association (MDA), July 15, 2005. Available online.

Plasmapheresis

URL: www.mda.org/sites/default/files/publications/Facts_Plasmapheresis_P-206_0.pdf. Accessed March 12, 2024.

Heitz, David. "Plasmapheresis: What to Expect," Healthline, September 3, 2018. Available online. URL: www.healthline.com/health/plasmapheresis. Accessed March 12, 2024.

"Plasma Exchange (Plasmapheresis) for MS," *Web*MD, August 16, 2023. Available online. URL: www.webmd.com/multiple-sclerosis/plasma-exchange-ms. Accessed March 12, 2024.

"Plasmapheresis and Plasma Exchange," Cleveland Clinic, September 20, 2022. Available online. URL: https://my.clevelandclinic.org/health/treatments/24197-plasmapheresis-plasma-exchange. Accessed March 13, 2024.

Stieglitz, Elliot; and Huang, James. "Plasmapheresis Technique," Medscape, January 25, 2023. Available online. URL: https://emedicine.medscape.com/article/1895577-technique?icd=login_success_gg_match_norm&isSocialFTC=true. Accessed March 12, 2024.

Chapter 29 | Vitamin D Therapy for Multiple Sclerosis

In recent years, there has been an accumulation of evidence that suggests vitamin D may have a role in preventing the occurrence of multiple sclerosis (MS) and perhaps in the treatment of the disease. Vitamin D is a fat-soluble vitamin. It is ingested in the diet as a precursor form and is normally converted to an active form by a process that involves chemical reactions triggered by ultraviolet light produced by the sun and by enzymes that are primarily produced by liver and kidney cells but also by immune cells. A product of this reaction is 25-hydroxy vitamin D, which can be measured in blood to determine whether a person has normal levels or is deficient in vitamin D.

The primary effects of vitamin D had been ascribed to the maintenance of bone health. However, it is now apparent that the vitamin also has important effects on the function of the immune system. With respect to MS, vitamin D deficiency has been linked with an increased risk of developing the disease. This was initially shown in a study performed in a cohort of nurses in which it was found that an increased intake of vitamin D, either in the diet or in the form of supplements, was associated with a lower risk of MS. The results of this study were supported by the findings of a subsequent study in which analysis of blood samples from military personnel showed that individuals who had the highest levels of vitamin D had the lowest risk of developing the disease, and the risk increased with progressively lower levels of vitamin D.

Subsequently, a large number of studies have provided further information regarding the effects of vitamin D in MS. These include evidence that higher vitamin D levels are associated with lower numbers of new lesions as well as less brain atrophy on magnetic resonance imaging (MRI). Higher vitamin D levels were not clearly associated with a lower chance of relapses, but people with MS were found to be less likely to develop worse disability. Such information suggests that vitamin D supplementation would likely result in people obtaining such beneficial effects. Unfortunately, so far it has not been demonstrated from clinical trials that taking vitamin D supplements, which can be purchased over the counter, can have a beneficial effect on a person's course of MS. It has been found from such studies, however, that supplementation can have effects of immune function in a manner that can be expected to be beneficial to people with MS.

There are many potential reasons why it has been difficult so far to show a definite benefit from taking vitamin D supplements in MS. These include the fact that there is strong evidence for benefit from vitamin D in MS and with respect to overall health, so it is difficult to ethically justify a clinical trial where one of the study groups is given placebo instead of vitamin D. Also, for people who are in a clinical trial, it is difficult to monitor the amount of vitamin D that is otherwise being ingested in the diet since there are many sources of the vitamin in addition to its availability as a supplement.

Finally, we have learned from studies that involved currently approved MS drugs that clinical trials that are designed to study potential MS therapies require larger numbers of people than what have been enrolled in vitamin D treatment trials to date. It can be difficult to enroll the required number of people for such studies. However, there are randomized, controlled clinical trials that are currently planned or underway that will examine larger numbers of people. These studies will also formally examine specific questions such as the effects of a higher versus a lower dose of vitamin D and whether such doses are safe and well tolerated. Observation studies in which people were not randomized to take a particular treatment suggest that vitamin D can be effective when it is administered in

Vitamin D Therapy for Multiple Sclerosis

combination with one of the U.S. Food and Drug Administration (FDA) approved disease-modifying therapies. This will also be studied in a clinical trial in which people will be randomly assigned to take a specific dose of vitamin D with their standard MS drug.

As we await information from these studies, people with MS are advised to take vitamin D supplements and have their vitamin D levels checked at regular intervals. The daily dose of vitamin D that will be optimal for people to take will be learned from clinical trials. It is currently recommended that the average person take up to 2,000 international units (IU) of vitamin D in combination with 1,000–1,200 milligrams (mg) of calcium. Low calcium levels impede the body's normal use of vitamin D and can promote a false increase in vitamin D levels.

However, common recommended doses of vitamin D in people with MS are between 1,000 and 4,000 IU of vitamin D_3 per day, with individuals treated with doses within this range being very unlikely to develop complications related to toxicity from taking the vitamin. It is possible to check blood levels of 25-hydroxy vitamin D and to use the result as a guide for how much vitamin D should be taken. The normal range for 25-hydroxy vitamin D level in blood is 30–74 nanograms per milliliter (ng/ml). Levels between 20 and 30 ng/ml are referred to as insufficient, and vitamin D deficiency is defined as levels less than 20 ng/ml.

People with MS should discuss their vitamin D levels with their health-care provider, including testing and approaches to ensure adequate levels. Additional information related to vitamin D and MS can be found on the websites of the National MS Society (www.nationalmssociety.org/Living-Well-With-MS/Diet-Exercise-Healthy-Behaviors/Diet-Nutrition/Omega-3) and National Institutes of Health Office of Dietary Supplements (https://ods.od.nih.gov/factsheets/VitaminD-Consumer).[1]

---

[1] "Update on Vitamin D," U.S. Department of Veterans Affairs (VA), November 15, 2022. Available online. URL: www.va.gov/MS/TREATING_MS/Whole_Health/Update_on_Vitamin_D.asp. Accessed February 22, 2024.

Chapter 30 | Stem Cell Therapy for Multiple Sclerosis

Stem cell therapy is an experimental procedure being studied in multiple sclerosis (MS) as a way to "reset" the immune system so that it is less likely to attack myelin. Since the first human studies in 1995, stem cell therapy has shown great potential for preventing MS disease activity but with risks of serious complications. Ongoing studies are trying to determine which people with MS will benefit most from stem cell therapy, and which stem cell therapy methods are safest and most effective.

Studies of stem cell therapy for MS generally use a type of stem cell therapy called "autologous hematopoietic stem cell therapy" (aHSCT). Autologous means the stem cells used for treatment are taken from the treated person's own body. Hematopoietic stem cells (HSCs) are adult stem cells found in bone marrow and blood which are capable of producing all of the cells that make up the blood and immune system. The process of aHSCT starts with medications that release stem cells from the bone marrow into the blood. These stem cells are then collected and frozen. This is followed by a treatment course of chemotherapy to suppress the remaining immune system. Finally, the previously collected stem cells are infused back into the patient's blood.

This one-time process usually takes place in the hospital over several weeks. An analysis of 15 individual studies on aHSCT in MS found that five years after the procedure, between 59 and 70 percent of people had no evidence of MS disease activity, while the combined mortality (death) rate from the procedure was 2.3 percent. Further analysis of this data showed that those with relapsing-remitting MS had better outcomes and safety compared to those with progressive MS. Importantly, the newer trials had lower rates of complications, further evidence that more time and experience with these procedures increases the safety.

In recent years, there has also been an increasing number of for-profit and nonaccredited stem cell treatment centers offering this procedure as well as increasing "stem-cell tourism" where people travel to other countries to receive stem cell therapy.

Still unknown is how effective aHSCT is at treating MS compared to some of the most effective MS therapies such as natalizumab (Tysabri), ocrelizumab (Ocrevus), and alemtuzumab (Lemtrada). The best available therapy versus autologous hematopoietic stem cell transplant for MS (BEAT-MS) study, currently ongoing at multiple sites across the United States, will help answer this question as well as further study the safety of aHSCT in people with aggressive MS who are not responding optimally to available MS medications.[1]

The most common form of MS is relapsing-remitting MS (RRMS), which affects about 80 percent of people with the disease. It is characterized by periods of mild or no symptoms interspersed with periods of more severe symptoms, called "relapses." It can change into a progressive form where symptoms worsen over time without any symptom-free periods. RRMS can be treated with drugs that suppress the immune system and reduce inflammation. However, these drugs can cause serious side effects, are costly, and patients may become resistant to them over time.

One promising treatment for MS is high-dose immunosuppressive therapy with autologous hematopoietic cell transplant (HDIT/HCT). The goal of this therapy is to "reset" a person's immune system so that it will stop attacking their central nervous system (CNS). The treatment involves first collecting a patient's hematopoietic stem cells (HSCs)—precursor cells that develop into

---

[1] "Stem Cell Therapy for Multiple Sclerosis," U.S. Department of Veterans Affairs (VA), February 13, 2024. Available online. URL: www.va.gov/MS/TREATING_MS/Whole_Health/Stem_Cell_Therapy.asp. Accessed February 23, 2024.

Stem Cell Therapy for Multiple Sclerosis

blood cells. High-dose chemotherapy and other drugs are then used to deplete the immune system and remove disease-causing cells. Finally, the participant is infused with his or her own HSCs, which develop into red and white blood cells and reestablish their immune system.[2]

---

[2] "Stem Cell Transplant Induces Multiple Sclerosis Remission," National Institutes of Health (NIH), February 14, 2017. Available online. URL: www.nih.gov/news-events/nih-research-matters/stem-cell-transplant-induces-multiple-sclerosis-remission. Accessed April 25, 2024.

Chapter 31 | Halting Multiple Sclerosis Progression

IMMUNE SYSTEM RESET TO HALT MULTIPLE SCLEROSIS PROGRESSION

Multiple sclerosis (MS) is an autoimmune disease in which the immune system attacks the central nervous system (CNS). It results in damage to nerve fibers, disrupting communication between the brain and the body. The disease's widely varying symptoms can include tingling or numbness in extremities, motor and speech difficulties, weakness, fatigue, chronic pain, vision loss, and depression.

The most common form of MS is relapsing-remitting MS (RRMS), in which periods of mild or no symptoms are interspersed with periods of more severe symptoms, called "relapses." RRMS can change into a progressive form where symptoms worsen over time without any symptom-free periods. RRMS can be treated with medications that suppress the immune system and reduce inflammation. However, these drugs can cause serious side effects.

One promising treatment for MS is high-dose immunosuppressive therapy (HDIT)/autologous hematopoietic cell transplant (aHCT). The goal of this treatment is to "reset" the immune system so that it will cease attacking the CNS. First, a patient's hematopoietic stem cells (HSCs)—precursor cells that develop into blood cells—are collected. High-dose chemotherapy and other drugs are then used to deplete the patient's immune system. Finally, the patient is infused with his or her own HSCs, which develop into RBCs and WBCs to reestablish the patient's immune system.

Past clinical trials have suggested that HDIT/aHCT may not work in patients with later-stage, progressive MS who already show marked neurodegeneration. However, the approach might be effective in patients with early-stage RRMS. Researchers from across the country are monitoring 24 volunteers with RRMS for five years following HDIT/HCT treatment. The clinical trial is funded by the National Institute of Allergy and Infectious Diseases (NIAID) of the National Institutes of Health (NIH). Interim three-year findings appeared online on December 29, 2014, in the *JAMA Neurology*.

Three years after HDIT/aHCT treatment, nearly 80 percent of trial participants had survived without an increase in disability, relapse of MS symptoms, or new brain lesions. Patients did not receive any MS drugs during those three years. Few serious early complications or unexpected side effects occurred. Many participants experienced issues that typically accompany high-dose immunosuppressive therapy, such as infections and gastrointestinal problems.

"These promising results support the need for future studies to further evaluate the benefits and risks of HDIT/HCT and directly compare this treatment strategy to current MS therapies," says the National Institute of Allergy and Infectious Diseases (NIAID) Director Dr. Anthony S. Fauci.

The researchers plan to follow participants for a total of five years. Final results from this and similar studies will help inform the design of larger trials to further evaluate HDIT/aHCT in people with MS.[1]

IDENTIFYING AND CORRECTING VITAMIN D INSUFFICIENCY TO HALT MULTIPLE SCLEROSIS PROGRESSION

Among people with early-stage MS, those with higher blood levels of vitamin D had better outcomes during five years of follow-up. Identifying and correcting vitamin D insufficiency could aid in

---

[1] News and Events, "Immune System Reset May Halt Multiple Sclerosis Progression," National Institutes of Health (NIH), January 12, 2015. Available online. URL: www.nih.gov/news-events/nih-research-matters/immune-system-reset-may-halt-multiple-sclerosis-progression. Accessed February 22, 2024.

Halting Multiple Sclerosis Progression

the early treatment of MS. People who have low levels of vitamin D intake or low blood levels of vitamin D have a higher risk for MS. This suggests that vitamin D is related to the disease, but it is unclear whether low vitamin D levels are a cause or a consequence of MS. An international team of researchers, led by Dr. Alberto Ascherio of Harvard School of Public Health, found that higher serum 25(OH)D levels in the first 12 months predicted reduced MS activity and a slower rate of MS progression. By the end of the follow-up at five years, participants with serum 25(OH)D concentrations of at least 50 nmol/L (20 ng/mL, a moderate level) had significantly fewer new active lesions, a slower increase in brain lesion volume, lower loss of brain volume, and lower disability than those with serum 25(OH)D concentrations below 50 nmol/L. These results suggest that vitamin D has a protective effect on the disease process underlying MS.[2]

---

[2] "Vitamin D Levels Predict Multiple Sclerosis Progression," National Institutes of Health (NIH), February 3, 2014. Available online. URL: www.nih.gov/news-events/nih-research-matters/vitamin-d-levels-predict-multiple-sclerosis-progression. Accessed April 25, 2024.

Chapter 32 | Complementary Approach for Multiple Sclerosis

Wellness is about physical, emotional, spiritual, and psychological well-being. Staying well with multiple sclerosis (MS) means not just keeping on top of your MS but also taking charge of your general health. Staying well may require you to take a holistic look at the many areas of life that can affect your health—your work environment, relationships, diet, sleep patterns, and more.

Being healthy and well is much more than making the symptoms go away.[1]

THUNDER GOD VINE IN THE TREATMENT OF MULTIPLE SCLEROSIS
- Thunder god vine, also known as "lei gong teng," is a perennial commonly grown in Southeast China. It has reportedly been used for hundreds of years in traditional Chinese medicine (TCM).
- Currently, thunder god vine is promoted for use orally (by mouth) for MS, rheumatoid arthritis (RA), Crohn's disease, lupus, psoriasis, fever, and other conditions.
- The leaves and roots of thunder god vine are used.

---

[1] "Complementary Therapies and Multiple Sclerosis," U.S. Department of Veterans Affairs (VA), February 14, 2024. Available online. URL: www.va.gov/MS/TREATING_MS/Complementary_Therapies.asp. Accessed February 23, 2024.

Multiple Sclerosis Sourcebook, Third Edition

What Have We Learned?
- Preliminary research suggests that oral or topical thunder god vine might be beneficial for RA symptoms. Some studies have suggested that thunder god vine plus standard medical treatment may be more effective than standard treatment alone for symptoms such as joint swelling and tenderness. Other studies have suggested that thunder god vine on its own may be at least as effective as standard medical treatments in reducing joint swelling and tenderness.
- A small amount of preliminary research suggests that thunder god vine might be helpful for Crohn's disease, some kidney disorders, and psoriasis, but there are no definite conclusions.
- There is not enough evidence to show whether the thunder god vine is helpful for other health conditions.

What Do We Know about Safety?
- Thunder god vine may have side effects, including digestive problems, abnormal heart rates, high blood pressure, less blood cell production, kidney problems, decreased bone mineral content (with long-term use), infertility, menstrual cycle changes, rashes, diarrhea, headache, and hair loss. Because some of these side effects are serious, the risks of using thunder god vine may be greater than its benefits.
- It can be extremely poisonous if the extract is not prepared properly.
- Thunder god vine should not be used during pregnancy because it may cause birth defects. Little is known about whether it is safe to use thunder god vine while breastfeeding.

Complementary Approach for Multiple Sclerosis

Keep in Mind
- Thunder god vine should not be used to replace conventional medical care.
- Take charge of your health—talk with your health-care providers about any complementary health approaches you use. Together, you can make shared, well-informed decisions.[2]

---

[2] "Thunder God Vine," National Center for Complementary and Integrative Health (NCCIH), January 2021. Available online. URL: www.nccih.nih.gov/health/thunder-god-vine. Accessed February 23, 2024.

Chapter 33 | Rehabilitation Options for People with Multiple Sclerosis

Rehabilitation medicine describes efforts to improve function and minimize impairment related to activities that have been hampered by disease, injuries, or developmental disorders.

Multiple sclerosis (MS) is a condition that may cause or contribute to disability. The primary effects of MS are physical—perhaps mobility or sensory problems. But individuals facing them can also experience intellectual, behavioral, and communication difficulties. They might have problems with making decisions, paying attention, or speaking. These can also require rehabilitation medical care.

WHAT TYPES OF ACTIVITIES ARE INVOLVED WITH REHABILITATION MEDICINE?

Rehabilitation medicine uses many kinds of assistance, therapies, and devices to improve function. The type of rehabilitation a person receives depends on the condition causing impairment, the bodily function that is affected, and the severity of the impairment. The following are some common types of rehabilitation:

- **Cognitive rehabilitation therapy (CRT).** This involves relearning or improving skills, such as thinking, learning, memory, planning, and decision-making that may have been lost or affected by brain injury.
- **Occupational therapy.** This therapy helps a person carry out daily life tasks and activities in the home, workplace, and community.

- **Physical therapy.** This involves activities and exercises to improve the body's movements, sensations, strength, and balance.
- **Rehabilitative/assistive technology.** This technology refers to tools, equipment, and products that help people with disabilities move and function. This technology includes (but is not limited to):
  - orthotics, which are devices that aim to improve movement and prevent contracture in the upper and lower limbs (For instance, pads inserted into a shoe, specially fitted shoes, or ankle or leg braces can improve a person's ability to walk. Hand splints and arm braces can help the upper limbs remain supple and unclenched after a spinal cord injury.)
  - wheelchairs, walkers, crutches, and other mobility aids
  - augmentative/alternative communication (AAC) devices, which aim to either make a person's communication more understandable or take the place of a communication method (They can include electronic devices, speech-generating devices, and picture boards.)
  - telemedicine and telerehab technologies, which are devices or software to deliver care or monitor conditions in the home or community
  - rehabilitation robotics
  - mobile apps to assist with speech/communication, anxiety/stress, memory, and other functions or symptoms
- **Recreational therapy.** This therapy helps improve symptoms and social and emotional well-being through arts and crafts, games, relaxation training, and animal-assisted therapy.
- **Speech and language therapy.** This aims to improve impaired swallowing and movement of the mouth and tongue, as well as difficulties with the voice, language, and talking.

Rehabilitation Options for People with Multiple Sclerosis

- **Vocational rehabilitation.** This aids in building skills for going to school or working at a job.
- **Music or art therapy.** This therapy can specifically aid in helping people express emotion, in helping cognitive development, or in helping to develop social connectedness.

These services are provided by a number of different health-care providers and specialists, including (but not limited to):
- physiatrists (also called "rehabilitation physicians")
- occupational therapists
- physical therapists
- cognitive rehabilitation therapists
- gait and clinical movement specialist
- rehabilitation technologists
- speech therapists
- orthopedists/surgeons
- neurologists
- psychiatrists/psychologists
- biomedical engineers
- rehabilitation engineers

The goal of rehabilitation medicine is twofold:
- to maximize function, participation, independence, and quality of life (QOL) for a person with a disabling condition
- to maintain and prevent any further decline in a person's functioning[1]

---

[1] "Rehabilitation Medicine," *Eunice Kennedy Shriver* National Institute of Child Health and Human Development (NICHD), January 14, 2022. Available online. URL: www.nichd.nih.gov/health/topics/rehabilitation-medicine. Accessed February 23, 2024.

Part 4 | Living with Multiple Sclerosis

Chapter 34 | Optimizing Life with Multiple Sclerosis

People with multiple sclerosis (MS) want to know what they can do today to feel their best, and if lifestyle interventions, such as diet, stress management, and physical activity, have any benefits in reducing the effect of the disease. Over the years, the concept of health has evolved to include a dynamic sense of well-being across multiple dimensions of life.

Wellness is attainable for everyone, even when living with a chronic illness. Achieving health and wellness is a lifelong process in which people make intentional choices, set personal priorities, and engage in health-promoting activities. Intentional choices include choosing the foods you eat, choosing whether to smoke, choosing to spend time with friends and family, choosing to engage in physical activity, devoting time to intellectual stimulation, and more.

Making healthy choices that promote satisfaction in the various dimensions of wellness can help you attain a sense of well-being and life satisfaction. The dimensions of wellness include the following:

- **Physical**. Making positive lifestyle choices about regular movement geared to one's abilities (such as walking, swimming, and yoga), healthy eating, regular engagement with one's health-care team, and preventive health behaviors (including smoking cessation, limited alcohol use, and attention to personal safety).

- **Social.** Developing positive, healthy relationships that nurture connections with family, friends, and community.
- **Emotional.** Developing coping strategies to enhance problem-solving, manage stress, foster a positive outlook, and develop resilience in the face of unpredictable changes, while paying attention to mood changes, such as depression and anxiety, that may require treatment.
- **Occupational.** Engaging in meaningful and rewarding activities that promote a sense of purpose and accomplishment, including opportunities to contribute one's unique skills, talents, and knowledge to others at home, at work, or in the community.
- **Spiritual.** Developing a worldview that provides a sense of peace and harmony, enabling one to cope and adapt throughout life—with the ultimate goal of finding meaning and purpose in the face of one's personal challenges.
- **Intellectual.** Engaging in mentally stimulating and challenging activities that lead to personal growth, enhanced creativity, and new learning.

As people manage their MS, they want to understand the role of conventional medicine, including disease-modifying therapies and symptom management medications, as well as how they can integrate lifestyle interventions and complementary approaches to maximize their well-being. They may wonder about the effect of a specific diet or exercise regime on MS or about the potential benefit (or harm) of other approaches such as vitamin supplements, probiotics, or acupuncture. Many have felt frustrated by a lack of support from health-care professionals, who say there is not sufficient scientific evidence to provide guidance, or who may not have the time or expertise to discuss it with their patients.

While many things may feel beyond one's control when living with an unpredictable and chronic disease such as MS, exerting control over your personal lifestyle behaviors can help alleviate feelings of helplessness. Setting your own personal wellness objectives and discussing them with your health-care providers are the first steps to maximizing your well-being. Some tips for incorporating wellness behaviors into everyday life include the following:

- **Make time to relax every day, even if only for 10–15 minutes.** Listen to music, utilize breathing techniques, or listen to a guided relaxation meditation.
- **Consider making a small healthy change or addition to your diet.** Replace dessert with a piece of fruit twice per week, try a new vegetable once per week.
- **Explore yoga, tai chi, or another physical activity.** It can be modified for your level of ability and interest.
- **Make a plan to regularly enjoy time with friends or family.** Watch a movie together, enjoy a meal together, or take a walk together.
- **Listen to an audiobook, attend a lecture, take an online course, and visit the museum.** Stimulate your curiosity and enhance your intellectual well-being.

Resources about wellness and MS, including information about diets that have been explored for MS, exercise and physical activity, mindfulness, and other strategies can be found at www.nationalmssociety.org/Living-Well-With-MS. For additional information about MS, please contact the National MS Society at (800) 344-4867.[1]

---

[1] "Living Your Best Life with Multiple Sclerosis," U.S. Department of Veterans Affairs (VA), February 13, 2024. Available online. URL: www.va.gov/MS/TREATING_MS/Whole_Health/Living_Your_Best_Life_with_Multiple_Sclerosis.asp. Accessed February 26, 2024.

Chapter 35 | Building Resilience

People with multiple sclerosis (MS) may find that the physical, emotional, cognitive, psychological, and spiritual challenges of living with the disease can be overwhelming. Some may feel that the challenges of living with a chronic disease are very hard to face day after day. But many people living with chronic diseases, including MS, have learned that practicing behaviors that promote resilience is the secret to not just coping with the disease but thriving with it.

Resilience is commonly described as the ability to bounce back from difficult circumstances—to find happiness and life satisfaction despite challenges. These challenges can be with relationships, finances, health, or any of the myriad stressors that we face in life. It is finding hope and meaning in life, even while confronting obstacles. It is finding the motivation to take on new challenges and opportunities. It is thriving in the face of whatever life throws at you. Resilience is the ability to maintain or regain well-being and progress toward valued goals in the face of adversity.

Resilience is not about acting happy all the time or ignoring the very real difficulties in life. Resilience is not even about trying to eliminate negative thoughts or feelings. In fact, it is quite the opposite: A significant part of being resilient involves what researchers call "positive adaptation" or "realistic optimism"—remaining hopeful about the future while making plans that enable us to cope with our actual reality. It requires moving forward despite facing difficult events and emotions. It requires courage and hope.

Results of several studies suggest that people who are resilient report significantly greater satisfaction with their lives. A study in the *Journal of Health Psychology* evaluated 1,862 people with MS, muscular dystrophy, post-polio syndrome, or spinal cord injuries. The researchers used various tests to assess the participants' resilience, including levels of depression, pain, fatigue, and overall quality of life (QOL). The study team found that people with higher resilience scores also had lower rates of depression and a higher QOL, even if they had high levels of pain and fatigue.

Other studies suggest that when people engage in activities that boost resilience, for example, stress management, social activities, or exercise, they report greater life satisfaction. Some people may be more naturally resilient than others. Researchers have found that people have a natural "set point" for resilience that is determined partly by genetics and partly by their early environmental circumstances. Together, those factors make up about half of a person's capacity to adapt positively to significant challenges. The other half of resilience comes from learning and using cognitive, behavioral, and interpersonal skills. Even if it does not come entirely naturally, you can learn to be more resilient.

Dawn Ehde, PhD, a psychologist at the University of Washington, collaborated with the National MS Society and MS Society of Canada to create a video and workbook about resilience. The workbook describes three steps to building resilience:

- **Understanding**. Learn as much as you can about MS and how it can change over time. Talk to others living with this chronic disease.
- **Managing**. Use your knowledge to learn new ways to cope and live your life with MS, with physical, social, and financial adjustments. You may feel more confident and in charge.
- **Growth**. Begin to shift your priorities and determine what is most important in life.

There are also lifestyle practices that can help people develop resilience:

- **Maintain strong social connections**. Family, friends, and others who have MS.
- **Maximize physical wellness**. Healthy eating habits, exercise, sleep, and MS therapies.

Building Resilience

- **Set realistic goals and move toward them.** Attainable goals result in feelings of competence.
- **Practice gratitude.** Be mindful of positive things in life.
- **Nurture positive emotions and savor them when they occur.** Hope, optimism, and humor.
- **Allow negative feelings.** Recognize, express, and move on.
- **Use mindfulness and relaxation approaches.** Develop techniques to reduce worry.
- **Practice forgiveness toward people and situations.** Release resentment and bitterness.
- **Plan for the future.** Make realistic assessments and practical adjustments.
- **Find a sense of meaning and purpose in life.** Relationships, activities, or other avenues.
- **Help others.** Volunteer.
- **Turn to faith or spirituality.** Seek a larger sense of belonging and meaning in life.
- **Learn to tell a different version of your story.** Reframe it to see both sides.
- **Nurture your sense of humor.** Find humor in all sorts of experiences and benefit from more positive mental and physical health.

Rather than making a chore of your resilience-building activities, focus on the ones you really enjoy. Watching a movie with your friends or children builds resilience. So does having a hobby and taking time to enjoy it. Taking time to meditate or engage in mindful breathing can also boost your resilience. "It is within the vast majority of humans to become more resilient - to develop the hope that leads to feeling more happy or content," says Dr. Ehde.

"People with MS, perhaps more than most, can benefit from building their resilience because of the ongoing, unpredictable changes they face in their health, abilities, and self-image," notes

Dr. Ehde. "People who are resilient have the ability to grow from adversity. They can learn things about themselves, about what they value. They learn that they can get through tough things."[1]

---

[1] "Resilience: Addressing the Challenges of Multiple Sclerosis," U.S. Department of Veterans Affairs (VA), February 13, 2024. Available online. URL: www.va.gov/MS/TREATING_MS/Whole_Health/Resilience_Addressing_the_Challenges_of_Multiple_Sclerosis.asp. Accessed February 26, 2024.

Chapter 36 | Dietary Changes and Multiple Sclerosis

People with chronic diseases, such as multiple sclerosis (MS), often seek complementary therapies for their disease to help in ways that are otherwise not addressed by conventional treatment modalities. Diet can make people with MS feel that they can take charge of their disease. But how diet can influence MS is not yet clear. Emerging data suggests that diet may affect disability and symptoms such as fatigue in MS and may influence immune system function. Poor diet defined as not adhering to the U.S. Department of Agriculture (USDA) nutritional guidelines—is linked with an increased risk of developing MS.

Strong data also suggests an adverse relationship between obesity and MS, with obesity increasing the risk of neurologic disability in MS. Therefore, dietary change as a way to improve MS is an attractive notion.

SWANK DIET

One of the pioneers in understanding how diet affects MS was Roy L. Swank, MD, PhD. Very early on, Dr. Swank made observations about dietary differences in people with MS around the world. This led him to wonder if the foods that people with MS eat influence their MS symptoms or disease progression. This interest led to him developing a research study following a group of people with MS for a number of decades. As a new idea for the time, dietary changes for MS offered promise that different foods could favorably affect disability. Based on his studies, Dr. Swank promoted a low-fat diet, specifically with very low amounts of saturated fats (e.g., butter, cheese, and red meat) and polyunsaturated oils (plant-based).

WAHLS PROTOCOL

Dr. Terry Wahls, a physician who had MS, devised a diet that was initially based on the idea that specific foods are better at providing key nutrients that maintain neurologic function. This idea has evolved into specific recommendations based on limiting certain dietary components such as lectins (a specific kind of naturally occurring protein found in most plants) that are thought to promote intestinal permeability and nervous system inflammation. In addition, Dr. Wahls has developed a form of therapy to accompany the diet that includes electrical stimulation of muscles. Despite gaining plenty of attention, clinical trials to evaluate the effect of the Wahls Protocol are still being completed.

FASTING

Many cultures and religions practice fasting, sometimes in part for health benefits. Modern medical studies suggest intermittent fasting may favorably influence various health conditions, including cancer, heart disease, and autoimmunity. Intermittent fasting can take many different forms, all of which are designed to cycle between low energy consumption and nonfasting conditions.

A very interesting research study, led by Dr. Laura Piccio of Washington University in St. Louis, Missouri, is exploring the effects of intermittent fasting on neurologic disability in MS. Specifically, the study aims to examine how changes in the diet of people with MS may affect the type of bacteria in their intestines. This link between diet and the bacteria in the intestines, part of the so-called microbiome, is an area of intense focus. Studies in this area could eventually lead to skipping any dietary changes by instead consuming specific "helpful" bacteria as a supplement (known as a "microbiome transplant") to improve neurologic function in people with MS.

KETOGENIC DIET

Other diets helpful for common diseases could also have benefits for MS. One of these is the ketogenic diet. When the body relies primarily on fats rather than carbohydrates for energy, ketone bodies are produced. Ketogenic diets have been employed as one strategy to treat epilepsy for many decades. In preliminary research, people with relapsing-remitting MS showed physical and mental improvement on a ketogenic diet. Additional studies are clearly needed and have been set in motion.

HOW TO CHANGE YOUR DIET

A key ingredient in making dietary changes for health purposes is not only which diet to use but also how to stick to it. Changes in diet are truly a lifestyle modification and require a strong commitment. Many approaches to assist with diet changes are being developed, including commercial applications. For example, one company combines monitoring certain physical and behavioral patterns with immediate and strict nutritional guidance to keep people on a ketogenic diet to help manage diabetes. Making a long-term, meaningful lifestyle change can certainly be very difficult. It is possible that in the near future using a phone or watch application could make these lifestyle changes simpler.

As hard as it is to change your diet, it is also challenging to study how dietary modifications can influence MS. One important component is also having the right support by the family members as they are also going to be involved. It is very different from just taking a pill!

Overall, there are several important points to consider about diet and MS. First, there is probably no one best diet for all people with MS. At this time, there is not enough scientific evidence to recommend a specific diet for people with MS. Second, diet alone does not appear to be a substitute for disease-modifying therapy prescribed to help reduce relapse rate and accumulation of MS disability over the course of disease. Third, diet is important to overall well-being, so consideration of dietary changes for MS need to take into account the health of each individual. Fourth, if you want to improve your health by changing your lifestyle, you should consider not only improving your diet but also adopting a healthy exercise regimen. Finally, changing your diet can be hard but even small improvements may be helpful.[1]

---

[1] "Dietary Changes for People with Multiple Sclerosis," U.S. Department of Veterans Affairs (VA), February 13, 2024. Available online. URL: www.va.gov/MS/TREATING_MS/Whole_Health/Dietary_Changes_for_People_with_Multiple_Sclerosis.asp. Accessed February 26, 2024.

Chapter 37 | Exercise Guidelines for Multiple Sclerosis

Chapter Contents
Section 37.1—Creating Your Activity Plan and
　　　　　　Exercise Routine...213
Section 37.2—Tips for Effective Exercise..................................218

Section 37.1 | Creating Your Activity Plan and Exercise Routine

Learning the best way to exercise after developing a life-changing disease such as multiple sclerosis (MS) can be challenging.

WHY IS EXERCISE IMPORTANT?

Exercise is important for a number of reasons. Exercise can help minimize some general health diseases such as cardiac disease and diabetes (as well as others) that can affect people with or without MS. It is also important in helping to minimize the effect of some of the problems that MS causes, such as weakness. If you can maintain your strength and ability to move about, then you are going to minimize the effect of some of the other problems.

People with MS are at risk of becoming deconditioned. Exercising and participating in a regular exercise program can help prevent this.

To prevent exercise from becoming boring, it should not be the same activity all the time. You should choose a variety of activities, but whatever you choose to do, you have to participate several times a week for exercise to help. To make it easier to exercise regularly, the most important thing is to schedule your exercise. By exercising regularly, you will learn more about yourself and become an expert in conserving energy, as well as become more efficient and thoughtful about how you are spending your time and energy.

WHAT TYPE OF EXERCISE IS BEST?

Health-care providers need to be aware of disease-specific issues when recommending exercise that is appropriate for people with MS. Fatigue is often a major issue when considering endurance or cardiovascular-type (aerobic) exercises and choosing an appropriate exercise plan can be a challenge. Typical methods of exercise for people with MS (as well as others) include walking, jogging, riding an exercise (or street) bicycle, or swimming.

If people are having difficulty walking, often a safe exercise program is using an exercise bicycle. The advantage of an exercise bicycle is that when people become fatigued, they are still at home and do not have to figure out how they are going to get home.

As MS progresses, it is common to have to shift to a different mode of exercise. Some people have to make this shift early on. They might have initially been joggers, and they no longer have the energy to keep jogging and need to explore other exercise options. Because it is easy to get into patterns and it is hard to change things on your own, it can help to have a professional evaluation.

HOW OFTEN SHOULD YOU EXERCISE?

It is generally recommended that people should exercise aerobically three to five times a week. This includes people with MS. As the goal, the duration of aerobic exercise should be 20 minutes or more of exercise each day. Unfortunately, because fatigue is a major MS symptom, starting out exercising at 20 minutes per session is usually not very realistic or possible.

Often people need to start out at three to five minutes at a time. Some will ask, "Is it even worth doing if I am only doing it three to five minutes?" The answer to this is that you have to start somewhere, so you start with what you can do and then you build on success, and build on success, and slowly increase your exercise time. Most people cannot jump 3–20 minutes in one exercise session. An alternate approach is trying two 10-minute sessions, which can be very beneficial.

The plan should be to start with three to four minutes, next increase from four to five minutes, and then from five to seven minutes, and so on. Remember, you can remain at those periods for as long as you need to until you are ready to go up to the next level. Exercising can help the psyche as well, and it is not just the physical aspects. Exercise endorphins, which are chemicals our bodies produce, that make us feel good are released during exercise. So there are physical and emotional benefits to exercising.

HOW HARD SHOULD YOU EXERCISE?

Some people find that MS causes numbness and tingling in the fingers, and it is hard to feel a heart rate. If this is an issue, it is generally recommended that you exercise to a level where a conversation can be held while still exercising. If you are having trouble carrying on a conversation, then you might be exercising a little bit too hard and need to slow down a bit. If you are able to converse without difficulty, then you probably are not exercising hard enough.

As you get stronger, you will want to increase the amount of exercise you do. One relatively painless way to get more exercise is to slowly increase the distance you park from a store (or other destination) each time you go. This will allow your body to strengthen itself while doing everyday chores. If you normally use a disabled parking pass, try parking in nondisabled spaces that are just a bit further away. You will find that you may be able to walk further as you gain strength. Of course, you can always use the disabled parking spot when you are trying to conserve your energy for the day.

This walking can be counted as exercise although a planned, structured exercise program is best. Keep in mind that unstructured exercise tends to wear you out, and then you are at risk for not being able to participate in an activity that might be more important to you later in the day.

Budgeting your energy is important. An example of budgeting your energy is if you have an important meeting at work, you might choose to park your car close to the entrance of the building to conserve your energy. If you need to be fully alert in the meeting, then you would want to conserve your "parking lot energy" for the energy that you will need for the business event. Walking a greater distance another day would make more sense.

People with MS need to be very careful about how they spend their energy and wisely choose their activities.

WHAT IS OVERHEATING WHEN EXERCISING?

When people with MS exercise—in fact when anyone exercises—they get warm. For people with MS, heat can be a big issue because it causes more fatigue. Doing strenuous exercise can be more of a problem for people with MS because often the ability to sweat—a body cooling mechanism—does not work normally. For some people, MS can affect the ability to properly sweat and to reduce overheating while exercising.

In fact, people with MS can become overheated with little to no exercise. For example, they can experience becoming overheated when out in the sun. There are a number of things you can do to help make up for the lack of (or reduction in) sweating that we do not typically think about. One method to prevent overheating is to dress in light clothing or layers of clothing that you can peel off as you warm up during the day. Another strategy is choosing to do your exercise in a cool room or environment to help with cooling your body down. If the rooms that you are living in are not cool, you might want to try to maintain a cooler temperature at least in the room where you exercise. Some people have used circulating fans to help cool their bodies during exercise. Having a cool beverage that you can take sips of now and then will really help keep you cool as well. If you swim as part of your exercise, try to swim in a pool that maintains a cooler temperature.

Another refreshing tip is to have a water spray bottle handy to spritz yourself as needed. In addition to helping you feel more comfortable, if you are someone who does not sweat normally (or enough), the spray/misting bottle will help provide artificial sweat and help cool your body down.

WHAT IS AN ACTIVITY DIARY?

Many people have found an activity diary to be a very useful tool. When you keep an activity diary for three to four days in a row (and during periods where you are doing regular activities), you start to see patterns of what you are doing. Once you see these patterns, you can change your activities so during your times of energy, you do activities that require energy and during your low energy times, you do things that do not take a lot of energy.

DO YOU NEED TO CHANGE YOUR ACTIVITIES?

When you get into a habit of doing things in a certain way, and then you get a diagnosis of MS, it forces you to do some things differently. It can be difficult to recognize that you have to change the way you do things. It can be difficult to change life habits, and that is where health-care professionals fit in—helping people through that process of change by directing them and showing them that there are different ways to do things. It is jarring enough to be diagnosed with MS, let alone all of the changes that are going to have to take place in one's life.

HOW DO YOU SET YOURSELF UP FOR SUCCESS?

When a person has decreased energy, setting goals, then prioritizing these goals is a very effective way of getting what is important done. Priority setting is typically based on the list of what needs to be done, what you would like to do, and what would be nice to do. The activities that are ticked off on any particular day are determined by the energy level of the day.

So how do you go about identifying what a goal ought to be? It should be something realistic, that you can achieve, and it should be specific. The more specific it is, the easier it is to tell if you have achieved it. It should also be something that can be done independently. You should not have to rely on other people to achieve this goal, and you should write it down, so you can review it regularly. One activity that should usually be included to help maintain function (even if it was not a habit before) is exercise.

CONCLUSION

Exercise can become part of your life with just a few modifications. You may want to consider asking your provider about a referral to a physical therapist for help developing an exercise program that is specific for you. Physical, occupational, and recreational therapists can help you design an appropriate program to help you "live with MS" more effectively.[1]

---

[1] "Planning Your Activities and Designing an Exercise Program," U.S. Department of Veterans Affairs (VA), February 13, 2024. Available online. URL: www.va.gov/MS/TREATING_MS/Whole_Health/Planning_Your_Activities_and_Designing_an_Exercise_Program.asp. Accessed February 26, 2024.

Section 37.2 | Tips for Effective Exercise

According to the National Center on Physical Activity and Disability: "In addition to improving overall health, cardiovascular fitness, range of motion, and flexibility, exercise can help one increase energy, improve balance, manage spasticity, decrease muscle atrophy, and better perform activities of daily living." Recent studies show that exercise is critical in preventing cognitive decline in those with multiple sclerosis (MS), central in lifting depression and overall mood and may even delay the progression of the disease. Below are six exercise tips for people with MS. Consult with your doctor before starting any exercise program.

1. STRETCH DAILY
Flexibility exercises, such as muscle stretching and range of motion exercises, can help prevent shrinkage or shortening of muscles and can help reduce the severity of spasticity symptoms. Dedicate at least 10–15 minutes of stretching every day, ideally several times a day.

2. EXPERIMENT
Multiple sclerosis affects everyone differently so try different ways of exercising to see what works best for you. Swimming and walking are popular, as are horseback riding and biking (try a three-wheeled trike if balance is an issue). Give a go at yoga, tai chi, or Pilates, or even an exercise class for older adults. Work out to videos at home or try circuit train at the gym. Adaptive ski programs can be a great way to enjoy the cool outdoors.

3. STAY COOL
Heat, while it will not trigger an attack, can exacerbate your MS symptoms, which can range from annoying to debilitating. Go to the gym when it is cool, exercise in the morning, seek out air-conditioning, consider snow sports, and put swimming (regardless

of how you look in a bathing suit) on your list. Use gear such as cooling vests and cold packs and do not forget to down icy drinks to keep your core temperature from rising too much.

4. CARDIO IS KEY

Multiple sclerosis research continues to support the importance of cardio workouts. Not only does it improve fatigue and overall quality of life (QOL) but also raising your heart rate appears to influence the progression of disease, decreasing both damage to the brain (fewer lesions) and brain atrophy. And yes, even if you are in a wheelchair, you likely can still do seated aerobic workouts.

5. TRAIN IN BURSTS

Fatigue or weakness can come on quickly, especially when doing the recommended cardio. Space out your "hard" exercise with frequent breaks if needed. High-intensity training, where you sprint for 10–30 seconds and then rest for a few minutes, can be quite effective. Mini workouts, all combined, produce the same or even better benefits as one long one.

6. REMEMBER, MULTIPLE SCLEROSIS MIGHT BE BEATABLE SOMEDAY

Multiple sclerosis might be beatable someday. Optimism when fighting an incurable disease is essential to good mental health. You want to be ready with the healthiest body and mind possible when a cure comes. You can definitely do this.[2]

---

[2] "Six Exercise Tips for Multiple Sclerosis," U.S. Department of Veterans Affairs (VA), February 13, 2024. Available online. URL: www.va.gov/MS/TREATING_MS/Whole_Health/Exercise_Tips_for_MS.asp. Accessed February 26, 2024.

Chapter 38 | Link Between Bladder Dysfunction and Falls in Multiple Sclerosis

Falls and bladder symptoms are common in people with multiple sclerosis (MS). More than 50 percent of people with MS fall in a three- to six-month period, and about 75 percent or more have problems with their bladder. It is now thought that in some people these symptoms may be related.[1]

The symptoms of bladder problems are wide ranging, and can include:
- **Urgency.** Barely getting to the bathroom in a timely manner.
- **Frequency.** Feeling the need to urinate more than every two to three hours.
- **Hesitancy.** Being unable to easily start a flow of urine.
- **Incontinence.** A loss of control of urine.
- **Nocturia.** Being awakened from a restful state by a need to urinate.
- **Double voiding.** Needing to urinate again a few minutes after voiding.

Other symptoms can be: feeling like the bladder is not empty after urinating, involuntary leaking of urine, difficult or painful discharge of urine, and urinary tract infections (UTIs).

---

[1] "Are Bladder Problems Tied to Falls in Multiple Sclerosis?" U.S. Department of Veterans Affairs (VA), April 1, 2021. Available online. URL: www.va.gov/MS/Veterans/research/Are_Bladder_Problems_Tied_to_Falls_in_Multiple_Sclerosis.asp. Accessed February 26, 2024.

Bladder symptoms are broken down into three basic types of problems: emptying problems (hypoactive bladder), storage problems (hyperactive bladder), and a mixture of these two types of problems (combined dysfunction). Each of these types of problems has a different treatment approach.[2]

A study led by Dr. Michelle Cameron, a neurologist at U.S. Department of Veterans Affairs (VA) Portland Healthcare System, VA MS Center of Excellence-West, found that in people with MS, urinary urgency (a sudden, compelling urge to urinate) with incontinence (involuntary leakage of urine) was associated with a significantly increased risk of falling multiple times in a three-month period. In fact, in this study, people who had both urinary urgency and incontinence had almost 60 times greater odds of recurrent falls compared to those people who did not have these bladder symptoms.

Interestingly, those people who only had urinary urgency or urinary frequency, but not incontinence, were not at increased risk for multiple falls. And no bladder symptoms were associated with an increased risk of just falling once.

Participants in this study had to meet certain criteria, including a confirmed diagnosis of MS, mild-to-moderate disability due to MS, no relapse within 30 days of the study start date, and be 18–50 years old to minimize the cause of falls being something other than MS. In addition, participants were excluded if they had balance or walking issues because of a condition other than MS, or if they could not walk at least 100 meters. In this study, a fall was defined as "any unexpected event that results in ending up on the ground, floor, or any lower surface." Of the 51 study participants, 32 people fell at least once in three months, and 15 fell at least twice in three months.

The findings of this study are important and useful because we really do not know all the reasons why people with MS fall or how to best help prevent them from falling so much. Many treatments to prevent falls in people with MS have been tried. Most of these consist of a combination of safety education and balance

---

[2] "Bladder Changes in Multiple Sclerosis," U.S. Department of Veterans Affairs (VA), February 13, 2024. Available online. URL: www.va.gov/MS/Veterans/symptoms_of_MS/Bladder_Changes_in_Multiple_Sclerosis.asp. Accessed April 30, 2024.

Link Between Bladder Dysfunction and Falls in Multiple Sclerosis

exercises. Although these may be helpful, they certainly do not fix the whole problem. They increase knowledge and improve people's balance, but they do not prevent all falls. Many of the reasons people with MS fall, such as weakness or numbness, probably cannot be fixed completely or easily. Finding that something such as urinary incontinence, which can often be treated easily and effectively with medications, may help prevent falls is, therefore, particularly encouraging. This study suggests that improved bladder management may be able to reduce the risk of falls in people with MS.

It is not clear why people with MS who have urinary urgency with incontinence tend to fall more. Although it is possible that they just have worse MS, this is not likely. In Dr. Cameron's study, statistical tests showed that the relationship between bladder symptoms and falls was not affected by how severe the person's MS was. So it is thought that bladder problems might cause falls in people with MS because, if you have urinary urgency and incontinence, you are likely to often rush to the bathroom, not paying as much attention to your safety when walking or transferring. It is also possible that people with bladder problems avoid drinking water and become dehydrated, which can then make them dizzy when walking.

If your MS affects your bladder, and you have frequent falls or near falls, tell your provider about it. Treatment for your bladder might not only help resolve or improve your bladder problems, but it might also help prevent you from falling.[3]

---

[3] See footnote [1].

Chapter 39 | Managing Bowel Issues

Bowel function is not something most people want to bring up in casual conversation. The topic might be uncomfortable or embarrassing, especially when things are not working as they should. But having a conversation about bowel function with your multiple sclerosis (MS) team is very important in helping you manage your symptoms and improve your function.

Most people with MS who experience bowel problems have constipation or report feeling "bound up" and have difficulty with regular bowel movements. The reason for this is related to your central nervous system (CNS), which is your brain and spinal cord. Together, the CNS speeds up or slows down the digestive process in your bowels. When the communication between your CNS and your bowels is disrupted, as it is in MS, the bowels tend to "slow down" and constipation can result.

Fortunately, there are many approaches and medications that can help with MS-related constipation. For some people with MS, managing their bowels is as straightforward as making time to have a bowel movement at the same time every day. This is best done after a meal because this is when your gut becomes more active and begins the digestion process. Sometimes people need more help with managing constipation, which is called a "bowel program."

Simply put, a bowel program is a combination of medications and routines that helps a person with MS-related constipation have bowel movements regularly and lessens the chance of incontinence or accidents. The first part of a successful bowel program is maintaining a regular, healthy diet, including consistent amounts of fruits, vegetables, and fiber, as these can affect how quickly or slowly your bowels move. Consultation with a registered dietician, a person who is trained to help people manage their diets to meet their health goals, can be valuable in managing your bowels. They can give you suggestions specific to your needs and situation that can help keep your bowels regular.

When diet changes alone are not enough, medications can be added to a bowel program. Medications for a bowel program tend to fall into one of two major types: oral or rectal. Oral medications are most commonly used. Oral medications might be in pill form or as a powder that is mixed with liquid that you drink. Oral medications can be taken by mouth or given through a feeding tube if a person with MS is unable to swallow. The goal of these medicines is to speed up bowels (a "stimulant") or to keep stools from becoming too hard (a "softener"). Some people may only need one type of oral bowel medication, while others may use a combination of several types.

While many people have success with oral medications alone, others might need rectal suppositories or enemas. A suppository is a round or cone-shaped medication that is put into the rectum or end of your intestine where stool exits. An enema is a liquid that is put into the rectum. The goal of both types of medications is to stimulate or speed up the bowels so that you have a bowel movement shortly after they are used. If an enema or suppository is needed, the time of day that it is given is important. The bowels are most likely to move after a meal, so most people use an enema or suppository after breakfast or dinner. While which time of day works best for a bowel program can be different for different people, being consistent with the time of day is important. Taking your medications at the same time each day improves your chances of success and makes accidents less likely over time. Think of it as "training" your bowels to move at a certain time each day and taking your medications as prescribed to match that time.

While constipation is the most common pattern of bowel dysfunction in people with MS, the opposite can also be true and bowel function can actually "speed up," causing loose stools, diarrhea, and incontinence. Sometimes loose stools are caused by foods in your diet. Common foods that can contribute to loose stools are spicy

Managing Bowel Issues

foods, fatty or fried foods, certain fruits high in a type of sugar called "fructose," and foods or drinks that have caffeine in them, such as chocolate, coffee, and alcohol. In this case, simply avoiding these foods can be helpful. Additionally, fiber can be helpful in making stools less loose.

Loose stools or diarrhea can also be caused by taking too many bowel medications. In that case, it is helpful to talk to your medical team about how to manage your medications to avoid loose stools while still having regular bowel movements and avoiding constipation. If this does not help, in some cases, other medications can also be prescribed to help slow down your bowels. However, you should talk to your provider before starting any over-the-counter medications to slow down your bowels because these can cause constipation if not used correctly.

While both constipation and loose stools can happen in people with MS, it is important to note if you have changes to your particular pattern. That is, if you usually have constipation and are now having loose stools, this can mean something else is causing it, or you are not on the right bowel program. Your health-care team can help you figure out the cause and make changes if needed.

In summary, while changes in bowel function related to MS may be frustrating or embarrassing to talk about, a conversation with your MS team is an important one to have. There is no "one-size-fits-all" solution to managing bowel function in MS but working closely with your providers can help you find a way to manage these issues in a way that works best with your life.[1]

---

[1] "Bowel Management in Multiple Sclerosis," U.S. Department of Veterans Affairs (VA), February 15, 2022. Available online. URL: www.va.gov/MS/Veterans/symptoms_of_MS/Bowel_Management_in_Multiple_Sclerosis.asp. Accessed February 26, 2024.

Chapter 40 | **Addressing Sexual Dysfunction**

Multiple sclerosis (MS) is a demyelinating disease which affects the central nervous system (CNS), causing a variety of problems such as fatigue, spasticity, muscle weakness, imbalance, altered bladder and bowel control, and sexual dysfunction. Sexual dysfunction is a common symptom in MS and affects more than 75 percent of people living with the disease; a frequency greater than that reported in other chronic diseases. Sexual dysfunction in MS has many causes.

IMPORTANCE OF ADDRESSING SEXUAL DYSFUNCTION

Sexual function is a vital element to a person's health and well-being. People living with MS are sexual beings, yet health-care providers often ignore or forget this part of a patient's identity. This avoidance to address and treat sexual dysfunction profoundly affects the quality of life (QOL) for all people living with MS; not only the person with MS but also his or her partner.

In reports of men with MS, sexual dysfunction may range 23–91 percent. Women may report sexual dysfunction up to 85 percent of the time. Eighty percent of the sexual dysfunction problems in men consist of erectile dysfunction (ED). In women, up to 72 percent report decreased libido and hyposexuality. Sexual dysfunction not only adversely affects QOL but also contributes to other problems as well. These problems can consist of:
- relationship conflict (marital problems noted in 71% of people with sexual dysfunction)
- depression, embarrassment, isolation, and despair

- performance anxiety
- avoidance and fear of intimate relationships and sexual encounters

Recognition of sexual dysfunction can help people with MS to:
- understand the problem
- lead to treatment
- build healthier relationships
- enhance self-esteem
- reduce depression
- promote patient-health-care provider relationships
- improve QOL

SEXUAL DYSFUNCTION MANAGEMENT

The first step in the management of sexual dysfunction is to acknowledge that sexual dysfunction is a significant health-care problem that most people with MS face at some point in their lives. It is also important to realize that sexual dysfunction is a subject that often goes under-recognized and under-treated. The second step is to talk about your sexual dysfunction concerns with your health-care provider. Physical therapists can address positioning techniques that enhance sexual comfort. Clinical psychologists can work with individuals or couples in promoting sexually sensitive communication to enhance sexual performance. Occupational therapists can instruct people in the use of sexual devices that can enhance sexual pleasure. Additional sexual dysfunction treatments may include the following:
- medical sex education materials
- oral medications (Viagra-sildenafil, Levitra-vardenafil, and Cialis-tadalafil)
- topical hormones
- sex therapy (body mapping other than genitals)
- counseling
- provision of sexual devices (vibrators, lubricants)
- intracorporeal injection of medication into the penis
- noninvasive physical treatments for ED (vacuum tumescence penis pumps)
- surgery for ED (implantation of inflatable or semirigid rods)

Addressing Sexual Dysfunction

Sexual dysfunction is a very prevalent problem in the MS population. It is a complex and dynamic interaction of physical, psychological, social, cognitive, and practical factors (financial). The person with MS, health-care team, and health-care community must work together to reduce sexual dysfunction if they hope to improve the QOL for all people living with MS.[1]

---

[1] "Sexual Dysfunction and Multiple Sclerosis," U.S. Department of Veterans Affairs (VA), February 13, 2024. Available online. URL: www.va.gov/MS/Veterans/symptoms_of_MS/Sexual_Dysfunction_and_Multiple_Sclerosis.asp. Accessed February 26, 2024.

Chapter 41 | Improving Sleep in Multiple Sclerosis

When you think of healthy habits for a healthy lifestyle, what is the first thing that comes to mind? If you are like most people, things such as healthy eating habits, exercise, or avoiding tobacco come to mind first. But what about sleep? More and more research is shedding light on just how important quality sleep is to our everyday lives. According to the National Sleep Foundation (NSF), poor sleep affects many parts of our health and our lives. People who do not get enough sleep are more likely to have problems with memory, concentration, learning, reasoning, weight, and a variety of serious health and mental health problems. The NSF estimates that about two-thirds of older adults suffer from sleep problems.

You have probably heard that as we age, we need less sleep, right? It turns out that this is a myth; our sleep needs to remain pretty constant throughout our adult lives. It is well-known and documented that people with multiple sclerosis (MS) have difficulty getting quality sleep consistently. From stiffness and rigidity to drowsiness from medications and rapid eye movement (REM) sleep behavior disorder, getting regular and quality sleep for people with MS can be very difficult. But what about the caregiver for the person with MS? How can he or she get better sleep? Below you will find some tips for good sleep hygiene that anyone can use to help make it more likely that you will get more quality sleep.

TIPS FOR GOOD SLEEP

- **Stick to a sleep routine/schedule.** Go to bed and get up at the same time each day, including weekends. Routine is

important; you want to train your mind/body with a good sleep routine.
- **Create a good sleeping environment.** No daytime activities in bed. This means no television (TV), eating, computer, or telephone. Train yourself to limit your bed-related activities, and your mind/body will "think" sleep in bed.
- **Relaxing ritual before sleep.** Reading, taking a bath, or listening to music—whatever it is for you, do something comforting and relaxing before sleep.
- **Avoid stimulants.** Generally speaking, you want to avoid caffeine three to four hours prior to sleep.
- **Limit food intake.** Avoid large meals or foods that cause indigestion prior to sleep.
- **Limit liquid intake.** Generally, avoid too much liquid intake three to four hours prior to sleep. This helps avoid having to get up due to nighttime urgency. This includes caffeine and alcohol.
- **Get some exercise.** Being physically active during the day can help you fall asleep more easily at night.
- **Bedroom temperature.** A cooler room is better for sleeping.
- **Naps.** Try to avoid naps later in the day. Generally speaking, no naps after 3 p.m.
- **Different beds.** Though this may not be the most appealing idea at first, you may want to try sleeping in a different bed than your spouse, particularly if your spouse acts out his or her dreams.[1]

It is important to practice good sleep habits, but if your sleep problems continue or if they interfere with how you feel or function during the day, you should talk to your doctor. Before visiting

---

[1] "Easy and Common Tips for Good Sleep," U.S. Department of Veterans Affairs (VA), February 13, 2024. Available online. URL: www.va.gov/MS/Veterans/symptoms_of_MS/Easy_and_Common_Tips_for_Good_Sleep.asp. Accessed February 26, 2024.

Improving Sleep in Multiple Sclerosis

your doctor, keep a diary of your sleep habits for about 10 days to discuss at the visit.

Include the following in your sleep diary, when you:
- go to bed
- go to sleep
- wake up
- get out of bed
- take naps
- exercise
- drink alcohol
- drink caffeinated beverages

Also, remember to mention if you are taking any medications (over-the-counter or prescription) or supplements. They may make it harder for you to sleep.[2]

---

[2] "What Do I Do If I Can't Sleep?" Centers for Disease Control and Prevention (CDC), September 14, 2022. Available online. URL: www.cdc.gov/sleep/about_sleep/cant_sleep.html. Accessed April 26, 2024.

Chapter 42 | Coping with Stress

Having multiple sclerosis (MS) can be incredibly stressful. Symptoms are unpredictable and can make it difficult to work, raise a family, or socialize; medications are expensive and come with a host of side effects. Many people report that stress aggravates their MS, and recent research confirms a connection between stress and worsening neurological symptoms. Thus, stress management is an essential component of a comprehensive MS treatment plan.

Many of the stressful situations we experience cannot be immediately changed (You probably cannot tell your in-laws that you are done spending holidays together or your kids to take a hike until they are 25.). If you cannot remove a specific stressor in your life, then the next best thing is to change your relationship to it, and meditation is one way to accomplish this.

WHAT IS MEDITATION?

Meditation is a mental exercise. It is common for people to think that meditation is about "clearing your mind" or creating a "blank mental slate," but this is not accurate. Meditation is actually a process of getting to know your mind. There are many different types of meditation. Some forms encourage participants to focus their attention on the breath, other forms suggest participants focus on a word or phrase that is repeated over and over, and still other types of meditation teach that the focus should be on one's internal experience: thoughts, feelings, and sensations.

While specific techniques may vary from one type to another, all meditative practices help cultivate self-observation, awareness, concentration, emotional regulation, and an attitude of acceptance. By practicing meditation, you can learn the patterns and habits of your mind, and then find new ways of approaching stressful life events that can lead to more satisfying and healthy experiences.

What Can Meditation Do for Me?

Regardless of the type of meditation, the general practice of focusing attention inward can induce changes in neural, immune, and endocrine function that lead to increased relaxation and improved physical and mental well-being. While research has yet to fully demonstrate how meditation effects change, studies have shown meditation can improve common MS symptoms, including fatigue, pain, sleep disturbance, depression, anxiety, and stress. More than just symptom management, meditation practice can empower participants by enhancing self-esteem, improving coping strategies, imparting a sense of control, and improving overall quality of life (QOL).

Meditation is a skill that must be practiced; the more you do it, the better the results. Like a muscle that needs exercise to become stronger, setting aside a few minutes each day to focus your attention will allow you to more readily access the physical and emotional benefits. Regular meditative practice will strengthen the neural connections associated with relaxation and emotional regulation, and with practice, you can access these connections in your day-to-day encounters with brief "meditative moments." Just a few focused breaths or a brief mindful reflection can create space between a stressful encounter and a habitual response, allowing your physiology (the way living things or any of their parts function) to shift and providing you more time for thoughtful action in a way that will help manage stress.

How Can You Get Started?

The demands of daily life are unlikely to disappear, but your response to these demands can change and that will in turn have a positive effect on your physiology. Commit to caring for yourself by making your stress-management plan as high a priority as

Coping with Stress

taking your medications or nutritional supplements. There are many resources out there so enjoy the exploratory process of finding a method that works for you and start crafting your own meditative practice today.[1]

COPING WITH POSTTRAUMATIC STRESS DISORDER

Multiple sclerosis is an unpredictable disease that is often accompanied by stress. Anxiety, depression, and other psychiatric problems are often experienced by people with MS. The rates of these problems in people with MS are higher than in those who do not have MS. People with psychiatric problems in connection with MS tend to report lower satisfaction with life. Additionally, studies show that psychiatric problems can result in worsening of MS disability.

While psychological and social stress is common in those with MS, some people also experience posttraumatic stress disorder (PTSD). PTSD is a disorder involving prolonged reaction in those who have undergone a scary or dangerous event. PTSD can be due to trauma from the battlefield, sexual assault, childhood abuse, or even due to a traumatizing medical diagnosis or procedure.

It is thought that PTSD and the stress related to it may potentially lead to additional neurochemical changes, leading to further inflammation, which leads to relapses and brain lesions. On the other hand, PTSD could lead to decreased adherence to MS medications. Given that psychiatric conditions associated with MS can lead to stress which can lead to worsened outcomes, strategies should be implemented to reduce stress. Coping is a behavioral strategy that can help to mitigate stress.

Art Therapy

One strategy for coping with MS-related stress is art therapy. While art as a form of therapy has been around for centuries, art therapy has become popular over the years to help people cope with chronic

---

[1] "Stress and Multiple Sclerosis: Can Meditation Help?" U.S. Department of Veterans Affairs (VA), February 13, 2024. Available online. URL: www.va.gov/MS/TREATING_MS/Whole_Health/Stress_and_Multiple_Sclerosis_Can_Meditation_Help.asp. Accessed February 26, 2024.

medical conditions. Artwork such as painting, writing, or creating music can help people with MS bring their stress and worries into the open, which can help to decrease the stress. Studies have shown that art therapy in those with MS can also help increase confidence and improve emotional well-being. Art therapy can also help those who are more disabled work on improved arm control.

Mindfulness

Another coping strategy shown to be useful is mindfulness. Mindfulness is defined as focusing on the present moment while understanding and accepting one's feelings, thoughts, and sensations. Practicing mindfulness originated in Eastern philosophy as a method for relaxation. Mindfulness has been shown to also help with managing anxiety, depression, and chronic pain. Classes in mindfulness can be taken and typically last around eight weeks. They tend to relate to different types of meditation such as being aware of the number and length of breaths being taken at a time, body awareness, and yoga.

Exercise

Exercise is another excellent way to cope. Exercises such as jogging, swimming, and using a stationary bicycle have been shown to be helpful for those with and without MS. Your health-care team, including the physical and occupational therapist, can help create a personalized program for you to address your specific abilities and needs. Another type of exercise worth seeking out is yoga. Yoga involves breathing and stretches that center on the spine. Depending on one's balance, changes can be made to ensure safety. Another similar exercise to yoga is tai chi, which is more "gentle." Tai chi also involves breathing, slow movement, and relaxation.

Pets

Finally, studies have shown that having a pet helps some people cope with a health problem. Being around pets can help take your mind away from dealing with the stress with MS. It can also help

Coping with Stress

with the stress of psychiatric conditions related to MS. A service pet is another option for those who need assistance with medical issues such as vision or walking. For those who do not want to own a pet, health-care programs are increasingly adopting a pet program where specially trained pets work with people.

These are just a few of the coping strategies of many that exist. Combining multiple coping skills can be ideal. Discussion of these coping strategies with your treatment team, including physicians, mental health providers, physical therapists, occupational therapists, and social workers, to optimize their effectiveness is essential.[2]

---

[2] "Coping Strategies for People with Multiple Sclerosis," U.S. Department of Veterans Affairs (VA), February 13, 2024. Available online. URL: www.va.gov/MS/TREATING_MS/Whole_Health/Coping_Strategies_for_People_with_MS.asp. Accessed February 26, 2024.

Chapter 43 | Fostering Effective Communication in Relationships

Multiple sclerosis (MS) is a chronic and unpredictable disease. A diagnosis of MS can affect every aspect of a person's life, including the relationship between partners and spouses. The uncertainty of MS can influence the daily routine or rhythms of life between partners, spouses, and other family members, and in turn, influence the lines of communication. Couples living with MS may often find it challenges their usual roles in the relationship and makes it hard to prioritize their relationship. Learning and practicing some simple, yet effective, communication and listening skills can foster a more supportive and intimate relationship while managing MS.

To facilitate and practice effective communication with a partner/spouse, identifying what may affect a relationship while living with MS can be explored together. For example, one partner may need to shift their work schedule to accommodate the other partner's medical appointments. Or one partner may need to juggle more of the household responsibilities while the other partner may need to scale back social activities. As roles and responsibilities shift, communication becomes even more essential to maintain a supportive relationship.

It takes time and energy to manage MS. The disease is often diagnosed in a person's most productive work years and can cause financial stress in couples. Financial management of a chronic disease, as well as the time and effort it takes to rethink tasks and routines, can affect communication. It is important for partners to talk about financial and legal planning to ensure that both individuals are prepared for a future with MS.

Although living with MS can have its challenges, it can also be an opportunity for growth in a couple's relationship. A life-altering diagnosis can bring a couple closer together, and foster more open, honest conversations, deepening mutual support and intimacy.

Following are the tips to help facilitate more open, positive, and supportive relationships.

COMMUNICATION TIPS FOR COUPLES

- **Make your relationship a priority by creating a culture of positivity.** Schedule "date" nights or couple time each and every week. Routine scheduled time for each other will allow for a foundation of positive communication to begin and blossom throughout the relationship.
- **Become an active listener.** Listening is 99 percent of communication. Give your partner all your attention and verbalize how important it is to listen to what is being said.
- **When listening to your partner, maintain good eye contact, let your partner finish speaking without interruption, and then ask for clarification if needed.** For example, "So, what I hear you saying is…". This helps ensure you and your partner are hearing and understanding each other.
- **Use "I" statements with your partner whenever possible.** For example, "I feel _____, when you help me bring in the groceries. Thank you." This clearly conveys your feeling of appreciation.
- **Keep in mind that effective communication skills need daily practice.** Pay attention to nonverbal communication such as body language and eye contact. And remember to be patient and open to growing together as a couple while learning to improve communication.
- **Maintain balance.** Identify ways by setting boundaries, scheduling time together that does not involve caretaking and ask for outside help as needed to help maintain roles within your relationship.

Fostering Effective Communication in Relationships

Sometimes couples may find they need more support and practice with their communication and listening skills.

People with MS can also contact their local U.S. Department of Veterans Affairs (VA) health-care facility and ask to speak with a social worker regarding options for family or couples counseling. If appropriate, your provider can refer you for couples counseling.[1]

---

[1] "Relationships: Improving the Lines of Communication," U.S. Department of Veterans Affairs (VA), November 15, 2022. Available online. URL: www.va.gov/MS/CAREGIVERS_PARTNERS/Improving_the_Lines_Of_Communication.asp. Accessed February 26, 2024.

Chapter 44 | Music Therapy for Multiple Sclerosis

The idea that music has a healing influence that can affect health and behavior has been recognized for centuries. The profession of music therapy formally began after World Wars I and II, when the therapeutic effects of music on physical and emotional traumas from the wars were recognized. From early studies in the 1800s, where psychologists used music to alter dreams for therapy, to currently using modern technology and equipment, the benefits of music therapy have become the focus of many organizations and discussion in journals worldwide.

IMPROVING MOVEMENT AND COORDINATION

The planning and order of movements are essential to everyday activity. Programs in which people learn to match repetitive motor actions (such as hand and foot exercises) with a computer-generated rhythmic beat can improve coordination, concentration, and physical endurance. Through these exercises, people experienced more even gait. Rhythm stimulates the impulse to move and helps people sidestep the coordination processes they cannot think through otherwise. It is almost impossible to fully lose the ability to process music because, unlike speech, it involves so many areas of the brain.

IMPROVING MEMORY

Memory changes are common in people with MS. Even though some people might find it difficult to recall particular pieces of information or to remember names, words, events, and so on, they can still learn to carry out new physical tasks. Studies show that the physical task of learning to play an instrument can improve cognition and memory. If long-term memories seem lost, some studies show listening to music might actually help those memories to return. This is because hearing music is associated with the areas of the brain where long-term memories are kept. As a result, listening to music from past special events or from "the good old times" in one's life can stimulate feelings and associations with those past events and in part improve access to long-term memories. Familiar music can also improve attention and memory recognition.

REDUCING DEPRESSION AND ANXIETY

Some of the hardest issues to cope with for people with MS are emotional ups and downs such as feelings of depression and anxiety. Expressing emotions by playing or listening to music can help some people cope with their past or present feelings and also help some deal with their fears. If music therapy is done in a group, it can help establish a closer connection with others, especially since music activates areas of the brain that process social signals, language, and emotions.

STRESS MANAGEMENT

Music can relax the mind and body and can even trigger physical reflexes, such as digestion, bladder control, and movement of the limbs. Mood may be enhanced by a particularly calming piece of music, and as a result, some people experience less discomfort or pain.

IMPROVED VERBAL COMMUNICATION

Music can also help people improve their verbal communication skills. Singing words that were otherwise difficult to recite has shown to aid in communication and verbal expression. For example, one might not be able to recite the words to "Happy Birthday," let alone speak fluently, but as soon as the words are set to music, the words can come naturally. Singing can also help with the breath support, pronunciation, and timing needed for speech.

Music Therapy for Multiple Sclerosis

Music therapy can help people with MS. It can help with depression, anxiety, memory, and other emotional issues. It also provides the physical benefits that come from staying active and moving. Healing through music, whether therapist-led or self-directed, can be an effective, low-risk, and low-cost endeavor.[1]

---

[1] "Music Therapy in Multiple Sclerosis," U.S. Department of Veterans Affairs (VA), February 13, 2024. Available online. URL: www.va.gov/MS/TREATING_MS/Whole_Health/Music_Therapy_in_Multiple_Sclerosis.asp. Accessed February 26, 2024.

Chapter 45 | Temperature Sensitivity in Multiple Sclerosis

People with multiple sclerosis (MS) often have a low tolerance for changes in their body temperature caused by air temperature, activity, digestion, or metabolic changes. Small increases—as little as ½ °F—in core body temperature can increase MS symptoms. Nerves that have lost their conductive coating (myelin sheath) become more sensitive to heat, and the nerve signal slows down or is blocked, resulting in an increase in symptoms. Depending on the location of the nerve damage in your body, symptoms may include increased heart rate, sweating, dizziness, muscle weakness, slowed reaction times, reduced energy, and difficulties with attention and concentration.

CAUSES OF INCREASED BODY HEAT
Many things can cause your body temperature to rise—some we usually think of, and some that are a little harder to see. Obvious causes of increased body temperature are things such as being in a warm environment, increasing physical activity, or wearing too many clothes. All these can easily lead to increased body temperature and an increase in MS symptoms. Less obvious causes of increased body heat include having a fever, changes in metabolism, hormonal changes, or side effects of medications.

Warm environments may include things such as your kitchen during meal preparation, working hard around your home (whether cleaning the house or working outdoors), taking a hot shower, swimming in a warm pool, or being out in the sun. Your body temperature may also rise with increased physical activity, such as when walking, propelling your wheelchair, exercising, or doing other leisure activities. Wearing clothing that keeps you too warm, or being in rooms that, although they are comfortable for others, are too warm for you may also increase your body temperature. Medical illnesses contributing to higher core body temperature may include bladder infections, colds, and the flu (causing a low-to-medium grade fever).[1]

Even young and healthy people can get sick from the heat if they participate in strenuous physical activities during hot weather:
- **Minimize outdoor exposure.** Limit your outdoor activity, especially midday when the sun is hottest.
- **Pace yourself.** Start activities slowly and pick up the pace gradually.
- **Drink more water than usual, and do not wait until you are thirsty to drink more.** Muscle cramping may be an early sign of heat-related illness.
- **Stay cool.** Wear lightweight, loose-fitting clothing.

If you play a sport that practices during hot weather, protect yourself and look out for your teammates:
- Schedule workouts and practices earlier or later in the day when the temperature is cooler.
- Monitor a teammate's condition and have someone do the same for you.
- Seek medical care right away if you or a teammate has symptoms of heat-related illness.

Everyone should take these steps to prevent heat-related illnesses, injuries, and death during hot weather:
- Stay in an air-conditioned indoor location as much as you can.
- Drink plenty of fluids even if you do not feel thirsty.

---

[1] "Keep Cool: Multiple Sclerosis and Heat Tolerance," U.S. Department of Veterans Affairs (VA), February 13, 2024. Available online. URL: www.va.gov/MS/TREATING_MS/Whole_Health/Keep_Cool_Multiple_Sclerosis_and_Heat_Tolerance.asp. Accessed February 26, 2024.

Temperature Sensitivity in Multiple Sclerosis

- Schedule outdoor activities carefully.
  - Wear lightweight, loose-fitting clothing, and sunscreen.
  - Pace yourself.
- Take cool showers or baths to cool down.
- Check on friends and neighbors and have someone check on you.
- Never leave children or pets in cars.
- Check the local news for health and safety updates.[2]

KEEPING COOL

If heat affects you, you need to take extra precautions and use strategies to keep cool. Minimizing your symptoms will help reduce the need for additional medications and maximize your independence and safety. There are several ways you can help your body to stay cool and keep yourself healthy.

Adjust the Temperature in Your Environment

- Use an air conditioner or fan in the room you are working in, or in your vehicle when traveling.
- Rest in rooms that are out of direct sunlight or have adequate shading over windows that have a western or southern exposure.
- When showering or bathing, turn the fan on in the bathroom and/or open a window if possible to help circulate the room air.
- Make sure the water temperature in your shower or bathtub is significantly lower than your body temperature and/or take a cool bath.
- Wear layered clothing that can be removed as necessary to adjust your body temperature.
- Avoid traveling to warm destinations during their hot and/or humid seasons.

---

[2] "Keep Your Cool in Hot Weather!" Centers for Disease Control and Prevention (CDC), September 12, 2023. Available online. URL: www.cdc.gov/nceh/features/extremeheat/index.html. Accessed April 26, 2024.

When you feel hot, use a spray bottle to mist yourself with water at regular intervals during activity (or even when sitting)—as many people with MS lose the ability to perspire and release body heat.

Drink Plenty of Fluids

During periods of increased activity, your body can generate several times the amount of heat it does at rest. The body releases excess heat by sweating and evaporation. Adequate water intake is important to be able to perspire during exercise and remain hydrated. Below are some tips for better hydration:

- **Place a plastic bottle of water in the freezer until frozen.** Put the bottle by your bedside at night so that you have cold water available to drink without having to get out of bed.
- **Stay cool and hydrated.** Drink chilled water, juices, and popsicles throughout the day to help keep your body temperature down.
- **Minimize caffeine for optimal cooling.** Avoid drinks with caffeine (e.g., sodas, colas, coffee, tea, chocolate, and some energy drinks). Caffeinated drinks are diuretics, causing you to lose fluid by increased urination. This leaves less fluid in your body to sweat (one of our natural ways of cooling down).

Use Cooling Equipment

- **Layer up with lightweight, breathable clothes.** Remove the layers as necessary to keep cool. Look for clothing that is designed to have more airflow through it, making it cooler to wear.
- **Shield yourself.** Use an umbrella while out in the sun.
- **Essential outdoor gear for sun safety.** Wear a vented hat, sunglasses, and use sunblock while outdoors. (The sunblock will not reflect heat but will help prevent you from skin cancer.)
- **Use a cooling vest.** Wearing a cool layer close to the skin effectively absorbs body heat to maintain a safe body temperature.
- **Use cooling packs on your wrists, neck, and on your head (under a hat).** Another strategy is to wear cloth-type

hats and dip them in water, allowing the sun to evaporate the water, cooling your head.

Develop a Personal Cooling Program

Research studies show that individuals who take a cool bath or shower (not cold), sit in an air-conditioned room, or wear a cooling vest for 45 minutes a day have an overall decrease in their core body temperature. This results in an improvement in strength and less fatigue for up to two hours after cooling. Below are some tips:
- Take a cool bath before working around the house or in the garden.
- Avoid hot or heavy meals, especially before going outside.
- Stay inside during the midday warmer hours.
- Take a shower in a swimsuit before working outside in it. The moisture in your suit will help cool you.
- Exercise or complete home management activities in the morning, the cooler time of the day.

COOLING VESTS

The above strategies work well for most people, but this does not mean that you will never have problems maintaining your body core temperature. When the "low-tech" methods (above) are not adequate, a cooling vest might meet your needs.

How Does a Cooling Vest Work?

A cooling vest is designed to keep the body's core temperature (around the heart and spinal cord) within safe levels to reduce symptoms of heat intolerance. The vest absorbs body heat, evaporates perspiration, and conducts cooler temperatures to the body through the skin. Cold packs for the neck, wrists, and head conduct cold through to the arteries, cooling the blood circulating in the body.

When Should You Wear a Cooling Vest?

The cooling vest should be worn in warm-to-hot conditions or when physical activity is planned. The vest can help keep you cool up to three hours when worn correctly although this can depend on things such as environmental temperature, humidity, and your level of activity.

How Do You Use the Cooling Vest?

It is beneficial to wear the cooling vest at least 30 minutes prior to physical activity. The cooling vest is more effective when worn over thin clothing and, when needed, when breathable fabrics are worn over the vest.

The vest usually has up to six Velcro closure pockets to house the cooling packs, two to four pockets on the front and three to four pockets on the back. Place each cooling pack into one of the pockets on the vest. Put the vest on and close the front. Adjust the side straps to provide a snug but comfortable fit with the cold packs in place.

Are There Different Types of Cooling Vests?

The following are different types of cooling vests that are recommended for people with MS:

- **Active cooling.** It requires an electricity source to operate the equipment that circulates air through the vest.
- **Passive cooling.** It is portable with no working components (e.g., gel inserts and ice packs, phase change—nonfreezing, cooling liquid in packs, embedded hydrogel crystals, and evaporative cooling—best in low humidity/arid environments).

How Do Traditional Cooling Pack Vests Work?

Initially, cooling packs should be put in the freezer overnight. Re-cooling them after use takes 30–60 minutes in the freezer. It does not harm the cooling packs to store them in the freezer. You will need to experiment to determine which level of cooling you can tolerate and is most beneficial to you. Some cooling vests have sleeves that cover the cooling packs and provide insulation. Layering clothing can help regulate the vest temperature to your comfort.

Temperature Sensitivity in Multiple Sclerosis

MANAGING TEMPERATURE SENSITIVITY ISSUES

If you are someone who has an increase in your MS symptoms when your body is overheated, it is important to use some of these methods to keep cool. If you experience heat intolerance, contact your medical team, which includes your primary care physician, neurologist, rehabilitation physician, or occupational therapist to find the best solution for your needs. They may provide adaptive equipment such as cooling vests to help you manage your symptoms.[3]

---

[3] See footnote [1].

Chapter 46 | Vaccinations for People with Multiple Sclerosis

Vaccines have been the focus of the news lately. Many questions come up when discussing the importance of vaccines for maintaining our health. Vaccines protect us from diseases without us having to experience the actual disease.

It is important to be up-to-date on your vaccinations before starting a disease modifying therapy (DMT) for your multiple sclerosis (MS). Fingolimod (Gilenya) might increase the risk of a potentially life-threatening varicella zoster virus (VZV) infections, so your provider will generally check for VZV antibodies before initiating fingolimod therapy. If immunity is not demonstrated by elevated VZV antibody levels, you will need the chicken pox (two-step) vaccination before starting fingolimod. It is recommended that you then wait one month after your last VZV immunization to let the vaccine work before starting fingolimod therapy.

FLU VACCINE
One of the most important vaccines is the influenza (flu) vaccine. Flu vaccines are important because flu is common, can be unpleasant, and can be fatal. The injectable flu vaccine has been studied extensively in people with MS and is considered safe for people getting a DMT for their MS. The flu vaccine is also available as an intranasal spray, Flu Mist, which should not be used in people with MS since it is a live vaccine. It is important to know that if a

family member receives this intranasal vaccine, they will shed the virus for up to one week after the vaccination. That means there is a possibility you can get the flu virus if you are exposed to their urine or feces during this period.

CHICKENPOX VACCINE

There are some people who have never had chickenpox or the chickenpox vaccine. Because fingolimod, alemtuzumab, and ocrelizumab can increase the risk of chickenpox in people with MS, if you are going to use fingolimod and have not had chickenpox or the vaccine, the Centers for Disease Control and Prevention (CDC) recommends that you receive the varicella vaccination. The varicella vaccine is given in two doses four weeks apart. People with MS should not start fingolimod until at least one month after the last dose of the varicella vaccine.

SHINGLES VACCINE

The Shingrix vaccine is a subunit vaccine, it provides part of the germ, that helps prevent shingles. Shingles is a painful outbreak of VZV, the same virus that causes chickenpox. Only a person who has previously had chickenpox can develop shingles. Shingles cause a painful rash and can result in persistent pain after the rash resolves. People with MS may be at higher risk of getting shingles because of reduced immune system function due to disease-modifying treatments. High-dose steroids, often used during relapses, may also increase the risk of a shingles outbreak. The Shingrix vaccine does not contain live virus and is safe for you to get. It is given by intramuscular injection requiring two injections, with the second dose given two to six months after the first.

PNEUMONIA VACCINE

The pneumonia vaccine (Pneumovax 23 and Prevnar 13) protects people from pneumonia caused by the pneumococcus bacteria. The difference in the two vaccines is how many types of bacteria they target. The vaccines are non-live, subunit vaccines. The pneumonia vaccine is recommended for people with compromised breathing or lung function, such as those who are wheelchair-dependent or bedbound because they are more prone to pneumonia. The CDC recommends that in order to acquire the best protection against all strains of bacteria that cause pneumonia, all adults 65 and older should receive the two pneumococcal vaccines. This vaccine is generally safe for people with MS.

HUMAN PAPILLOMAVIRUS VACCINE

This vaccine can prevent most cases of cervical cancer if given before a girl or woman is exposed to the virus. In addition, this vaccine can prevent vaginal and vulvar cancer in women and can prevent genital warts and anal cancer in women and men. The CDC recommends teens and young adults who begin the vaccine series later, at ages 15 through 26, continue to receive three doses of the vaccine. Additionally, the CDC recommends catch-up human papillomavirus (HPV) vaccinations for all people through the age of 26 who are not adequately vaccinated. The U.S. Food and Drug Administration (FDA) approved the use of Gardasil-9 for males and females aged 9–45.

COVID-19 VACCINE

Coronavirus disease (COVID-19) vaccines are an important component in preventing the spread of the COVID-19 virus. COVID-19 causes very serious illness and death, particularly to vulnerable people, including those who are older, immunocompromised, and have certain medical conditions. If you get COVID-19, you also risk giving it to loved ones who may get very sick. COVID-19 vaccines were tested in large clinical trials to make sure they met safety standards. It is not possible to get COVID-19 from getting the vaccination.

There are several types of COVID-19 vaccines. There is no chance that these vaccines change your deoxyribonucleic acid (DNA). Even after getting the vaccine, you should continue to wear a mask around others, wash your hands, and practice physical distancing to prevent the virus from "hopping" from you to others even when you do not get sick.

Overall, vaccines and their boosters are safe and effective for people with MS and should be utilized based on current guidelines. There are no concerns for use of non-live vaccines in people with MS. Live, attenuated vaccines should usually be avoided in people with MS when an effective, safe alternative is available. Vaccines should not be given during or within four to six weeks of an MS relapse. If you have any questions or concerns about vaccines, please talk with your health-care provider.[1]

HEPATITIS B VACCINE

Hundreds of millions of people worldwide have received hepatitis B (HepB) vaccine without developing MS or any other autoimmune disease. As with all vaccines and any disease, due to the large number of vaccinations administered worldwide, surveillance systems that monitor health concerns after vaccination do expect to receive reports of MS occurring after vaccination that happen by chance alone. To further explore any possible connection between HepB vaccination and MS, many scientific studies have been conducted, and have concluded that HepB vaccination does not cause MS.

Examples of this scientific evidence are:
- A study conducted in France from 1994 to 2003 compared children with MS to children without. The study did not find a relationship between vaccination for HepB and the development of childhood-onset MS.
- In the United States, a study compared 422 adults with demyelinating diseases, including MS, and 921 matched controls (people similar in age, gender, and enrollment in a health-care system, but who did not have demyelinating disease). The researchers concluded that HepB vaccination was not associated with demyelinating disease in the study population.
- Other studies conducted in the United States, Europe, and in British Columbia also evaluated the possible

---

[1] "Vaccines and Multiple Sclerosis: A Practical Guide," U.S. Department of Veterans Affairs (VA), February 13, 2024. Available online. URL: www.va.gov/MS/TREATING_MS/Whole_Health/Vaccines_and_Multiple_Sclerosis_A_Practical_Guide.asp. Accessed February 27, 2024.

Vaccinations for People with Multiple Sclerosis

   link between HepB vaccination and MS, and also found no association between HepB vaccination and MS.
- In 2002, the Institute of Medicine (IOM) reviewed published and unpublished research to determine if there was a link between HepB vaccine and demyelinating neurological disorders, including MS in adults. The committee found that the epidemiological evidence does not support a causal relationship between HepB vaccine in adults and MS.

CDC takes concerns about vaccines and immune system diseases and disorders very seriously. Researchers at CDC and elsewhere have conducted studies to examine the possible link between vaccines and autoimmune conditions like MS, diabetes, and asthma. These studies have been reassuring, providing no evidence to suggest a link between vaccines and autoimmune conditions.[2]

---

[2] "Hepatitis B Vaccine and Multiple Sclerosis FAQs," Centers for Disease Control and Prevention (CDC), August 20, 2020. Available online. URL: www.cdc.gov/vaccinesafety/concerns/history/hepb-faqs.html. Accessed April 22, 2024.

Chapter 47 | Dealing with Mobility Challenges

Mobility challenges can interfere with every aspect of everyday life. This can be true for people who are just beginning to experience difficulty with balance and walking, for those using walking aids such as canes or walkers and for those who use wheeled mobility to get around. Strategies to improve or maintain the ability to move around are certainly important. However, there are multiple other small changes people with MS can put into place that can have a big effect. This is one place where thinking small and taking it one step at a time can be effective.

HOW DO YOU BUDGET YOUR ENERGY?

A budget approach allows you to take charge of how you spend your energy and spend it on what matters most. Think about it in the same way as budgeting money. Begin by learning how to estimate the energy cost of different activities by noticing how tired you feel during and after those things that you do regularly. Keep in mind that fatigue is not just a result of spending physical energy. There can be cognitive and/or emotional energy costs that are just as important to consider.

Next, evaluate how much energy you have available. Then decide where you want to spend that energy—what activities do you consider to be the most essential, have the most value to you, or have a high priority for another reason? Consider if you can reduce energy costs by doing things in a different way (e.g., shopping online). Finally, you should plan your day or week, so you spend your energy on the things that matter most to you. Be proactive and decide what you want to drop, delegate to others, ask for help with, or move to another day or time to avoid "going in the red."

In MS, the amount of energy available can vary from day to day, or even within a day, for reasons that are not always obvious or predictable. Be prepared for these unexpected fluctuations by keeping some energy on reserve in your "energy bank" and having a backup plan that focuses on your highest priority activities.

HOW DO YOU PACE YOURSELF?

It can be tempting to rush to finish something before you get tired or to try to do just one more thing. However, with MS, it is critical to stop and rest before you start feeling tired. This may mean taking a "micro-break," stopping to sit for a few minutes before continuing with an activity or scheduling a regular nap or quiet time into your day. This can be hard to do when you feel like you have enough energy to keep going. However, not taking a rest before feeling tired can backfire and make you more fatigued in the long run.

WHAT IS YOUR POSITION?

You can use less energy by positioning objects and materials, so they are within easy reach. Store the objects you use most often in heights between shoulders and knees to minimize reaching and bending. Taking care of how you position yourself in relation to what you are doing can also reduce energy expenditure. Use the support of furniture (e.g., armrests) when you can and make sure you face the task directly. This uses less energy than working from a strained or awkward position. You can also sit on a chair or stool instead of standing to do some tasks. This includes tasks that are fairly quick, such as brushing your teeth in the morning, to those that take longer, such as washing the dishes. Put chairs or stools in those locations ahead of time to make it more likely that you will use them.

WHAT ARE ACTIVITY STATIONS?

Set up activity stations in your home to save steps and energy by putting the objects and materials used for a task together in one place. Activity stations can be for any routine task—getting dressed, making sandwiches, leaving the house, or washing the car. Start with something you do often. Get help as needed to move everything you use for that task to the place where it makes sense to do the bulk of the work. Then identify the things in that area that are not needed. Move the unneeded objects to where they will be used and either toss or give away the things you do not use on a regular basis. This approach can reduce not just your physical energy expenditure but also how much thinking is needed and emotional stress.

HOW CAN YOU MAKE LIFE EASIER?
Slide objects along countertops instead of lifting and carrying or use a utility cart to transport objects. Or save steps by using a transitional "staging area" when moving multiple items from one location to another, for example, when unloading the dishwasher or setting the table. Replace heavier objects and tools with ones that are more lightweight. Use tools and devices that increase leverage, such as a long-handled jar opener, or increase friction, such as a rubber gripper. Use electrical appliances and power tools stored within easy reach for both big and small jobs.

IS THERE ROOM TO GET AROUND?
It can be surprising how quickly clutter can accumulate. Clutter makes it more difficult to move around and can also make it more difficult to think clearly. Clearing out clutter is one way to give you enough room to get around safely. Moving furniture and electrical and phone cords out of the way is also helpful. Aim for clear, wide pathways with enough space for you and your mobility aid to move forward, change direction, and turn freely. If a narrow doorway is getting in your way, widen it by installing offset hinges. Most hardware and home supply stores carry this inexpensive solution.

HOW DO YOU KEEP THINGS "ON THE LEVEL?"
Make walking and standing surfaces safe, so there is nothing to trip over, slip on, or tip over. Flooring should be level with carpet

edges that are taped or tacked down. Get rid of loose rugs. If that is not an option, anchor them securely to the floor with tacks or tape. Door thresholds should be low-level with the floor is best. If needed, a mini threshold ramp can be installed.

HOW SUFFICIENT IS YOUR LIGHTING?

The goal here is sufficient lighting without glare. Aim for even lighting within and between rooms. Turn on the lights before you go into a room. If there is not a light switch within reach, move a lamp close to the entry or use night lights to make it easier to see where you are going. It is especially important to have enough lighting in areas such as entryways, hallways, and stairs and places, such as the bathroom, where you might be navigating at night.

DO YOU HAVE SOMETHING TO HOLD ONTO?

Adequate support can reduce the risk of falls. Install stair handrails on both sides of stairs, so you can hold on while going up and coming down. Use heavier furniture without caster wheels, so it will stay put when you sit down or stand up or position it against a wall to keep it in place. Transfer poles that go between the floor and ceiling are another option when there is not a place for a grab bar.

Falls in the bathroom often result in injury. This is not surprising given the hard, slippery surfaces, frequent need to move quickly, low heights, need to step over fixtures, and the possibility of overheating. A raised toilet seat can make it easier to get up and down from the toilet, or an over-the-toilet commode chair can provide additional support. Grab bars can make it safer to use the toilet and tub or shower, while nonskid mats or decals in the tub or shower can make those floors less slippery. A shower chair or a bench that goes over the edge of the tub, along with a hand-held shower nozzle, can make it possible to take a shower in a seated position when standing is more risky.

WILL YOU NEED A MAJOR REMODEL?

Many of the changes described here are relatively minor in scope and can be done with a "do-it-yourself" approach. However, when

Dealing with Mobility Challenges

faced with major remodeling and decisions about permanent changes, people with MS have found it helpful to "expect the best and prepare for the worst." This avoids having to go back and make costly changes later. Avoid person-specific solutions when possible and use universal design principles instead. These allow you to put solutions into place that work for everyone—you, your family, and guests in your home, as well as future buyers should you decide to move.

HOW DO YOU GET STARTED?

Time, energy, physical, and financial challenges can make it difficult to know where to begin. For most people, making or reviewing an energy management budget is a good first step. Then, look at the changes that give you the "biggest bang for your buck" and put those in place with the help of family, friends, and others in your support network. If you need more assistance with knowing what is best for you or how to go about making changes, a referral to an occupational therapist for additional guidance and specific suggestions may be helpful. While mobility challenges can seem overwhelming, taking one step at a time can make a difference.[1]

---

[1] "Meeting Mobility Challenges One Step at a Time," U.S. Department of Veterans Affairs (VA), February 13, 2024. Available online. URL: www.va.gov/MS/Veterans/symptoms_of_MS/Meeting_Mobility_Challenges_One_Step_at_a_Time.asp. Accessed February 27, 2024.

Chapter 48 | Features of Home Accessibility

People with multiple sclerosis (MS) become increasingly unable to take care of themselves. However, individuals will move through the disease in their own unique manner. The following general principles may be helpful.

- **Think prevention.** Even with the best-laid plans, accidents can happen. Therefore, checking the safety of your home will help you take control of some of the potential problems that may create hazardous situations.
- **Adapt the environment.** It is more effective to change the environment than to change most behaviors. You can make changes in an environment to decrease the hazards and stressors that accompany behavioral and functional changes.
- **Minimize danger.** By minimizing danger, you can maximize independence. A safe environment can be a less restrictive environment where the person with MS can experience increased security and more mobility.

HOME SAFETY ROOM-BY-ROOM

Prevention begins with a safety check of every room in your home. Use the following room-by-room checklist to alert you to potential hazards and to record any changes you need to make. You can buy products or gadgets necessary for home safety at stores carrying hardware, electronics, medical supplies, and children's items.

Keep in mind that it may not be necessary to make all the suggested changes. It covers a wide range of safety concerns that may arise, and some modifications may never be needed. It is important, however, to reevaluate home safety periodically as behavior and abilities change.

Your home is a personal and precious environment. As you go through the below list, some of the changes you make may influence your surroundings positively, and some may affect you in ways that may be inconvenient or undesirable. It is possible, however, to strike a balance. Caregivers can make adaptations that modify and simplify without severely disrupting the home. You may want to consider setting aside a special area for yourself, a space off-limits to anyone else and arranged exactly as you like. Everyone needs private, quiet time, and as a caregiver, this becomes especially crucial.

A safe home can be a less stressful home for the person with MS, the caregiver, and family members.

THROUGHOUT THE HOME

- **Keep essential numbers and home address handy.** Display emergency numbers and your home address near all telephones.
- **Use a telephone answering machine when you cannot answer calls.** The person with MS is often unable to take messages or may be a target for telephone exploitation by solicitors. When the answering machine is on, turn down the phone bell to avoid disruptive ringing.
- **Prioritize safety and maintain regular checks.** Install smoke alarms near all bedrooms; check their functioning and batteries frequently.
- **Avoid the use of flammable and volatile compounds near gas water heaters.** Do not store these materials in an area where a gas pilot light is used.
- **Enhance home security.** Install secure locks on all outside doors and windows.
- **Avoid the use of extension cords if possible by placing lamps and appliances close to electrical outlets.** Tack extension cords to the baseboards of a room to avoid tripping.

Features of Home Accessibility

- **Cover unused outlets with childproof plugs.** Covers protect your child from dangerous outlet tampering and electric shock.
- **Secure heating devices.** Place red tape around floor vents, radiators, and other heating devices to deter the person with MS from standing on or touching a hot grid.
- **Ensure proper illumination.** Check all rooms for adequate lighting.
- **Install light switches.** Place light switches at the top and the bottom of stairs.
- **Stairways should have at least one handrail that extends beyond the first and last steps.** If possible, stairways should be carpeted or have safety grip strips.
- **Each bottle of prescription medicine should be clearly labeled with the patient's name, name of the drug, drug strength, dosage frequency, and expiration date.** Child-resistant caps are available if needed.
- **Avoid clutter, which can create confusion and danger.** Throw out/recycle newspapers and magazines regularly. Keep all walk areas free of furniture.

OUTSIDE APPROACHES TO THE HOUSE

- Keep steps sturdy and textured to prevent falls in wet or icy weather.
- Mark the edges of steps with bright or reflective tape.
- Consider a ramp with handrails into the home rather than steps.
- Eliminate uneven surfaces or walkways, hoses, or other objects that may cause a person to trip.
- Place a small bench or table by the entry door to hold parcels while unlocking the door.
- Make sure outside lighting is adequate. Light sensors that turn on lights automatically as you approach the house are available and may be useful. They also may be used in other parts of the home.
- Prune bushes and foliage well away from walkways and doorways.

ENTRYWAY
- Remove scatter rugs and throw rugs.
- Use textured strips or nonskid wax on hardwood floors to prevent slipping.

KITCHEN
- Remove scatter rugs and foam pads from the floor.
- Remove knobs from the stove or install an automatic shutoff switch.
- Keep a night-light in the kitchen.
- Insert a drain trap in the kitchen sink to catch anything that may otherwise become lost or clog the plumbing.

BEDROOM
- Use a night-light.
- Use an intercom device (often used for infants) to alert you to any noises indicating falls or a need for help. This is also an effective device for bathrooms.
- Remove scatter rugs.
- Remove portable space heaters. If you use portable fans, be sure that objects cannot be placed in the blades.
- Be cautious when using electric mattress pads, electric blankets, electric sheets, and heating pads, all of which may cause burns. Keep controls out of reach.
- Move the bed against the wall for increased security or place the mattress on the floor.

BATHROOM
- Remove the lock from the bathroom door to prevent the person with MS from getting locked inside.
- Place nonskid adhesive strips, decals, or mats in the tub and shower. If the bathroom is uncarpeted, consider placing these strips next to the tub, toilet, and sink.
- Use washable wall-to-wall bathroom carpeting to prevent slipping on wet tile floors.

Features of Home Accessibility

- Use an extended toilet seat with handrails or install grab bars beside the toilet.
- Install grab bars in the tub/shower. A grab bar in contrasting color to the wall is easier to see.
- Use a foam rubber faucet cover (often used for small children) in the tub to prevent serious injury should the person with MS fall.
- Use plastic shower stools and a handheld showerhead to make bathing easier.
- In the shower, tub, and sink, use a single faucet that mixes hot and cold water to avoid burns.
- Adjust the water heater to 120 °F (48.89 °C) to avoid scalding tap water.
- Insert drain traps in sinks to catch small items that may be lost or flushed down the drain.
- Use a night-light.
- Remove small electrical appliances from the bathroom. Cover electrical outlets. If men use electric razors, have them use a mirror outside the bathroom to avoid water contact.

LIVING ROOM

- Clear all walk areas of electrical cords.
- Remove scatter rugs or throw rugs. Repair or replace the torn carpet.
- Place decals at eye level on sliding glass doors, picture windows, or furniture with large glass panels to identify the glass pane.
- Do not leave the person with MS alone with an open fire in the fireplace or consider alternative heating sources.[1]

---

[1] "Home Safety for People with Alzheimer's Disease," U.S. Government Publishing Office (GPO), 2002. Available online. URL: www.govinfo.gov/content/pkg/GOVPUB-HE20-PURL-LPS35559/pdf/GOVPUB-HE20-PURL-LPS35559.pdf. Accessed March 1, 2024.

Chapter 49 | Equipment for Self-Care and Independence

Many individuals who have multiple sclerosis (MS) begin to have difficulty with their mobility as the disease progresses. Changes in vision, decreased balance, increased spasticity, muscle weakness, changes in sensation, or a combination of these symptoms can affect mobility. When a decline in lower extremity function occurs, individuals may benefit from assistive devices, such as braces, canes, crutches, walkers, wheeled walkers, and manual wheelchairs.

WHEN DO YOU USE POWER MOBILITY?
There are several factors that should be considered when transitioning to power mobility. The first is your current functional status. You may be experiencing an increase in problems with your balance, near or actual falls because of muscle weakness and fatigue or other symptoms. You may also be having more difficulty completing self-care tasks and instrumental activities of daily living (home management, shopping, cooking, etc.) due to the additional effort it is taking to move around, keep your balance, and use assistive devices such as a walker or manual wheelchair.

Generalized fatigue, impaired fine motor function, and visual changes from the fatigue affect at least two-third of individuals with MS and also contribute to limitations in daily activities. While medications are available to combat primary fatigue in MS, many times secondary fatigue can be effectively managed by activity modification, energy conservation, balancing work and rest, and use of adaptive equipment. The goal of using power mobility is to maximize access to your home and the community, maintain safety, and conserve energy. Power mobility is an effective tool to reduce fatigue during daily activities by limiting the need for standing, reducing walking distances, and providing a method for "mobile" rest breaks during the day.

HOW DO YOU CHOOSE THE APPROPRIATE POWER MOBILITY DEVICE?

An individual assessment of mobility and function by an occupational or physical therapist will identify problem areas and lead to a stepwise intervention. The optimal outcome is a good match between your mobility needs and the power mobility device. The initial power mobility choice to be made is usually between a power scooter and a power wheelchair; selection between these two devices is based on your home environment, your functional status, and available transportation for the device.

It is very important to choose the best power mobility device to keep you as independent as possible in daily activities and assist with management of your symptoms, rather than a device that can be transported in any vehicle. With many advances in the design of power mobility devices and the large selection available, most of the time both the goal of remaining independent and transporting your device can be met.

WHAT ARE POWER SCOOTERS?

Individuals often first experience using a scooter at the local grocery or retail store. Scooters are three or four wheel power mobility devices that steer such as a bicycle using the tiller and are operated with both hands (either fingers or thumbs) controlling the forward and reverse levers. Scooters are intended for part-time use during the day despite having different options for seat size and back support. The seat can be turned next to a table in a restaurant to reduce the need for transfers, and attached baskets provide storage for shopping.

Equipment for Self-Care and Independence

Scooters range in weight from 80 pounds to over 250 pounds. Some can be disassembled and transported in a vehicle, however, frequently a vehicle lift is more desirable to reduce the work involved in getting around for daily living and community activities. Because of their design, scooters require a large area to turn around in and therefore are usually not useful inside the home.

To use a scooter safely, it is important that you have good trunk control, adequate upper body strength and dexterity to operate the controls, and the ability to transfer to/from the scooter seat.

WHAT ARE POWER WHEELCHAIRS?

If MS has affected your back and arm muscles, a power wheelchair may be needed to provide adequate support to maintain good posture, reduce fatigue, and prevent deformity. A power wheelchair is operated using a single hand, or other drive controls such as head movement. Because the batteries, motors, and drive wheels are directly under the seat, a power wheelchair has a much smaller turning radius which is helpful for in-home use and on public transportation.

There are numerous options to customize the seating system for help with transfers, reaching higher surfaces, independent pressure relief, and rest breaks. The primary disadvantage of a power wheelchair is its weight and inability to disassemble it for transport. Power wheelchairs range in weight from 200 to 500 pounds. Most private vehicles will require a vehicle lift to transport the device or an adapted van with a ramp or wheelchair lift.

POWER MOBILITY DEVICES FOR U.S. VETERANS

The process of obtaining power mobility within the U.S. Department of Veterans Affairs (VA) can take three to six months. While procedures may vary between VA facilities, most are similar in evaluating you, ordering the power mobility device, and then seeing you for follow-up. The VA has direct access scheduling, so if you would like to be evaluated for power mobility, you should contact your Rehabilitation or Spinal Cord Injuries and Disorders (SCI/D) scheduling department to schedule an appointment.

At your appointment, the clinician will evaluate you to determine the most appropriate mobility device for you and whether you meet VA medical eligibility criteria for power mobility. After eligibility is determined, the clinician will discuss power mobility options with you to find the "right fit" and order the device. Delivery of the scooter or power wheelchair can take 4–12 weeks depending on the complexity and customization of the device. Once the power mobility device is delivered, the clinician will schedule you for a follow-up appointment to adjust the seating, check the seat fit, and complete the initial training. Fit and training may require several sessions based on the complexity of the device and your familiarity with power mobility.[1]

Three primary factors for transporting power mobility are your physical ability to load a device (or availability of family/caregiver help), the type of power mobility device you own, and the type of vehicle you plan to use. Consider the following factors:

- How often will you use the scooter or power wheelchair—is using a manual wheelchair a better option?
- Will you need to purchase a different vehicle to make full use of your power wheelchair or scooter?
- How is your health, and/or how is the health of the person who will be loading and unloading your power mobility equipment?
- If you have a scooter and own a van, can you transfer to a van seat? (Please note: Riding on the scooter in a van is against safety regulations in many states.)
- If your vehicle cannot accommodate a lift and your power mobility device, will you or a care provider be able to disassemble/load/unload/assemble the device at each location you stop in the community?[2]

---

[1] "Power Mobility: Is It Time for Wheels?" U.S. Department of Veterans Affairs (VA), February 13, 2024. Available online. URL: www.va.gov/MS/Veterans/symptoms_of_MS/Power_Mobility_Is_it_Time_for_Wheels.asp. Accessed February 27, 2024.

[2] "Transporting a Scooter or Power Wheelchair," U.S. Department of Veterans Affairs (VA), February 13, 2024. Available online. URL: www.va.gov/MS/Veterans/symptoms_of_MS/Transporting_a_Scooter_or_Power_Wheelchair.asp. Accessed April 22, 2024.

Equipment for Self-Care and Independence

WHAT IS THE FOLLOW-UP PROGRAM FOR U.S. VETERANS?

Over time, if you experience further mobility limitations, it may be necessary to transition from a scooter to a power wheelchair or modify the current power wheelchair. It is important that you and/or your caregivers routinely monitor changes in your functional abilities such as upper extremity strength and dexterity, transfers, fatigue level, and driving safety to determine whether a follow-up appointment is needed.

The decision to use power mobility can be life-changing by giving you back the ability to access your indoor and outdoor environments. Although using a scooter or power wheelchair does not replace the need to exercise, it may improve your mobility and energy conservation for greater independence in daily living, work, and recreational activities.[3]

---

[3] See footnote [1].

Chapter 50 | Driving Considerations for People with Multiple Sclerosis

Driving is the most complex activity of daily living performed every day. It is important not to minimize the complexities of driving or overestimate one's abilities. Driving requires adequate vision, motor, memory, and thinking skills. Multiple sclerosis (MS) can affect all these areas. As MS evolves, required driving skills may diminish in several domains:

- blurred vision, poor night-time vision, blind spots, double vision, loss of color vision, impaired visual searching, scanning, and attention
- short-term memory loss, confusion about vehicle operation or one's location or destination, stress intolerance, impaired motor planning, multitasking, and reaction time, fatigue, and heat intolerance
- impaired sensorimotor function may manifest as difficulty with car transfers, muscle weakness or stiffness/spasms/cramps, poor light touch and joint position sensation, pain, and impaired coordination, particularly in the arms or feet

A cardinal feature of MS is its variability and unpredictability. Symptoms often fluctuate during the course of a day and from one day to the next. Most people with MS have a relapsing course and during exacerbations (attacks, relapses, or flare-ups), driving may be unsafe but may return to normal upon recovery. However, with disease progression, driving can become permanently affected.

If you, your loved ones, or your health-care provider are concerned about your driving ability, a driving evaluation performed by a driver rehabilitation specialist can help identify challenges you experience and the need for appropriate adaptive auto equipment to keep you safely on the road. The purpose of a driving evaluation is to assess driving skills, recommend adapted auto equipment if indicated to meet specific functional needs, and train the driver and family in its use, ensuring safety of entering/exiting the vehicle and proper storage of wheelchair and assistive devices.

The driver rehabilitation specialist makes recommendations on driving safety. Adapted equipment may be recommended. Examples include hand controls to operate the gas and brake, a spinner knob to help turn the steering wheel, power transfer seats, digital driving rings, and hi-tech driving equipment for reduced effort and zero effort steering and braking.

Keen awareness of the fluctuating nature of MS symptoms can help you avoid the risk of unsafe driving. Here are some tips:
- Do not drive if you are having a bad day.
- Avoid driving when you have another illness because MS symptoms are often worse when the "system" is under increased stress.
- Keep trips short if you suffer fatigue and do not drive when fatigue is severe.
- Avoid distractions such as cell phone calls/texting, eating, listening to the radio, and arguing with passengers.
- If you are heat intolerant, carry a cooling vest.
- Strategically plan out errands and appointments so that you can avoid heavy traffic times or areas that get congested.
- Avoid driving in bad weather.

WHAT IF YOU DECIDE TO STOP DRIVING OR ARE TOLD IT IS NO LONGER SAFE TO DRIVE?

Just as you plan for other circumstances associated with your disease (e.g., making your home more accessible), planning for the

Driving Considerations for People with Multiple Sclerosis

day when driving becomes impossible can ease the transition from driver to passenger. When transitioning from driver to passenger, explore transportation options in your community.

- Ask a friend, neighbor, or family member if they could give you a ride.
- Inquire about volunteer drivers at your local community center or place of worship.
- Contact your city and state public transportation agencies about transportation options.

Driving can be seen as a sign of independence, and it can be scary to think about limiting or giving up that freedom. A professional evaluation and the use of adaptive auto equipment can increase your safety on the road and promote independence for as long as it is safe for you to drive. If you feel like you can no longer safely drive, there are a variety of transportation alternatives and your family members, friends, and health-care professionals are here to help and support you with this transition.

Talking about how you feel may help you better understand and address the grief felt over these changes.[1]

---

[1] "Things to Consider about Driving," U.S. Department of Veterans Affairs (VA), February 13, 2024. Available online. URL: www.va.gov/MS/Veterans/symptoms_of_MS/Driving_and_Multiple_Sclerosis.asp. Accessed February 28, 2024.

Chapter 51 | Self-Advocacy and Effective Communication

Multiple sclerosis (MS) can be a life-changing diagnosis. The unpredictability of the disease may cause self-doubt and uncertainty about the future. The chronic, fluid, and ever-changing symptoms can affect the self-esteem and emotional wellness of many individuals living with MS. A sense of control and overall positive self-esteem and wellness can be regained through self-advocacy with ourselves, our loved ones, and the health-care community.

Self-advocacy can be translated into understanding your strengths and weaknesses, developing personal goals, being assertive (standing up for yourself), and making decisions that reflect your best interest. An effective self-advocate is someone who lets other people know what he or she is thinking, feeling, and needing. Self-advocacy does not mean someone will always get their desired outcome, but practicing the skills to self-advocate when living with a chronic illness can be an empowering, positive, and important step in living your fullest and healthiest life with MS.

Becoming a self-advocate while living with MS can allow others, such as family, friends, and health-care providers, to learn more about your unique perspective with managing MS symptoms. It can improve a sense of unity and belonging when advocating with others living with MS. It can increase awareness and educate loved ones, family, and friends about symptoms associated with MS that are not always openly discussed due to social stigma (such as bladder issues, cognitive changes, and depression). It can also empower and install a sense of hope and resiliency, which in turn promotes a positive feeling of overall wellness and direction. There are multiple strategies and various resources for becoming an effective self-advocate.

BELIEVE IN YOURSELF

You are valuable, unique, and worth the effort to advocate for your health-care needs. Know that your perspective is imperative in managing your MS wellness journey. Repeat the following affirmation each day to yourself, "I am worth the effort to self-advocate for my needs and be the healthiest person I can be."

SET GOALS FOR YOURSELF

Clarify what you need and use the SMART system to set goals that are Specific, Measurable, Achievable, Results-oriented, and Time-sensitive. For example, you may have difficulty remembering all the recommendations your health-care specialist provides for you during your visit. Or you may realize when you get home from a visit, that you are not sure where to start or what was said regarding a strategy for follow-up care. A SMART goal could be to ask your health-care specialist for a list of the recommendations, to get a printout of the follow-up instructions/health strategies, and to outline projected dates to complete any health tasks before your next appointment (e.g., blood work completed a week before returning to the clinic).

GET THE FACTS

- **Make sure you are armed with information that is accurate when advocating for yourself.** For example, if you feel you need to have a conversation about switching your disease modifying therapy (DMT) with your MS provider, make sure you do your due diligence in finding unbiased information about each DMT option.
- **Gather support.** Nothing helps self-advocacy more than supportive family and friends. Educating family members

Self-Advocacy and Effective Communication

and friends on MS and rallying the troops when you need support can be a great confidence builder and lessen feelings of isolation.

COMMUNICATE AND EXPRESS YOUR NEEDS CLEARLY

Learning how to communicate effectively takes some practice, but with a SMART plan in place, you can begin to develop good communication skills. If you feel like you may forget a point, or lose your train of thought, write it down or record your thoughts ahead of time. Be firm, but do not lose your temper, if you find you have resistance from family, friends, or community organizations when self-advocating. Listen to what the other person is trying to communicate to you. Be persistent in advocating for what you need while remaining open to a compromise to move forward.

It may take several tries before you feel more confident in expressing yourself in a concise, clear, and direct manner, but practice does make perfect when advocating for yourself.[1]

---

[1] "Communication Matters: Self-Advocacy," U.S. Department of Veterans Affairs (VA), February 13, 2024. Available online. URL: www.va.gov/MS/TREATING_MS/Whole_Health/Communication_Matters_Self_Advocacy.asp. Accessed February 27, 2024.

Part 5 | Multiple Sclerosis, Work, Financial, and Legal Issues

Chapter 52 | Accommodating Employees with Multiple Sclerosis

People with multiple sclerosis (MS) may develop some of the limitations discussed below, but seldom develop all of them. Also, the degree of limitation will vary among individuals. Be aware that not all people with MS will need accommodations to perform their jobs, and many others may only need a few accommodations. The following is only a sample of the possibilities available. Numerous other accommodation solutions may exist.

QUESTIONS TO CONSIDER
- What limitations is the employee with MS experiencing?
- How do these limitations affect the employee and the employee's job performance?
- What specific job tasks are problematic as a result of these limitations?
- What accommodations are available to reduce or eliminate these problems? Are all possible resources being used to determine possible accommodations?
- Has the employee with MS been consulted regarding possible accommodations?
- Once accommodations are in place, would it be useful to meet with the employee with MS to evaluate the

effectiveness of the accommodations and to determine whether additional accommodations are needed?
- Do supervisory personnel and employees need training regarding MS?

ACCOMMODATION IDEAS
Activities of Daily Living
- Allow use of a personal attendant at work.
- Allow use of a service animal at work.
- Make sure the facility is accessible.
- Move workstation closer to the restroom.
- Allow longer breaks.
- Refer to appropriate community services.

Cognitive Impairment
- Provide written job instructions when possible.
- Prioritize job assignments.
- Allow flexible work hours.
- Allow periodic rest breaks to reorient.
- Provide memory aids, such as schedulers or organizers.
- Minimize distractions.
- Allow a self-paced workload.
- Reduce job stress.
- Provide more structure.

Fatigue/Weakness
- Reduce or eliminate physical exertion and workplace stress.
- Schedule periodic rest breaks away from the workstation.
- Allow a flexible work schedule and flexible use of leave time.
- Allow work from home.
- Implement ergonomic workstation design.
- Provide a scooter or other mobility aid if walking cannot be reduced.

Accommodating Employees with Multiple Sclerosis

Fine Motor Impairment
- Implement ergonomic workstation design.
- Provide alternative computer access.
- Provide alternative telephone access.
- Provide arm supports.
- Provide writing and grip aids.
- Provide a page turner and a book holder.
- Provide a notetaker.

Gross Motor Impairment
- Modify the worksite to make it accessible.
- Provide parking close to the worksite.
- Provide an accessible entrance.
- Install automatic door openers.
- Provide an accessible restroom and break room.
- Provide an accessible route of travel to other work areas used by the employee.
- Modify the workstation to make it accessible.
- Adjust desk height if wheelchair or scooter is used.
- Make sure materials and equipment are within reach range.
- Move workstation close to other work areas, office equipment, and break rooms.

Heat Sensitivity
- Reduce worksite temperature.
- Use a cool vest or other cooling clothing.
- Use a fan/air conditioner at the workstation.
- Allow flexible scheduling and flexible use of leave time.
- Allow work from home during hot weather.
- Provide speech amplification, speech enhancement, or other communication device.
- Use written communication, such as email or fax.
- Transfer to a position that does not require a lot of communication.
- Allow periodic rest breaks.

Vision Impairment
- Magnify written material using hand/stand/optical magnifiers.
- Provide large print material or screen reading software.
- Control glare by adding a glare screen to the computer.
- Install proper office lighting.
- Allow frequent rest breaks.

SITUATIONS AND SOLUTIONS

A claims representative for a government agency was having difficulty reading files due to vision impairment caused by MS. His employer purchased a stand magnifier and added task lighting to his workstation.

A manager with MS working for a publishing company was having difficulty transferring from her wheelchair to the toilet in the employee restroom. Her employer installed additional grab bars.

An attorney with MS was having difficulty carrying documents to meetings at various locations due to upper extremity weakness. His employer purchased a portable cart that was easy to get into and out of his car.

An operations clerk for a large distribution center was having difficulty working at full production due to fatigue caused by MS. Her employer moved her to a shift that was not as busy so caused less stress and made less physical demands of the clerk. The clerk was also able to take more frequent breaks on the new shift.

An engineer with MS was experiencing heat sensitivity. She was provided a private office where the temperature could be lower than in the rest of the facility. She was also encouraged to communicate with coworkers by telephone or email when possible to reduce the amount of walking she had to do.

A resource nurse with MS was having difficulty accessing her workstation. Her employer widened the floor space in her workstation to allow her easier access from her wheelchair and added an adjustable keyboard tray, monitor holder, and telephone tray. In addition, the employee was provided a flexible schedule, so she could continue her medical treatment.

Accommodating Employees with Multiple Sclerosis

A clerical worker was having difficulty concentrating and remembering job tasks due to cognitive impairment caused by MS. Her employer added sound baffle panels to reduce distractions in her work area. In addition, her employer gave her written job duties at the beginning of each day and provided a notebook that contained outlines of what each job duty entailed.

A teacher with MS was having difficulty communicating with students because his speech became soft and slurred when he was fatigued. He was given a personal speech amplifier, so he would not have to strain to project his voice, and he was allowed to schedule his classes so he could take periodic breaks.[1]

---

[1] Office of Disability Employment Policy (ODEP) "Accommodation and Compliance Series," U.S. Department of Labor (DOL), March 23, 2010. Available online. URL: www.govinfo.gov/content/pkg/GOVPUB-L41-PURL-gpo9235/pdf/GOVPUB-L41-PURL-gpo9235.pdf. Accessed February 28, 2024.

Chapter 53 | Disability Benefits for Multiple Sclerosis

Disability is something most people do not like to think about. But the chances that you will become disabled are probably greater than you realize. Studies show that a 20-year-old worker has a one in four chance of becoming disabled before reaching full retirement age. The disability benefits are provided through two programs: the Social Security Disability Insurance (SSDI) program and the Supplemental Security Income (SSI) program.

WHO CAN GET SOCIAL SECURITY DISABILITY BENEFITS?

Social Security pays benefits to people who cannot work because they have a medical condition that is expected to last for at least one year or result in death. Federal law requires this very strict definition of disability. While some programs give money to people with partial disability or short-term disability, Social Security does not. Certain family members of disabled workers can also receive money from Social Security.

HOW DO YOU MEET THE EARNINGS REQUIREMENT FOR DISABILITY BENEFITS?

In general, to get disability benefits, you must meet two different earnings tests:
1. A recent work test, based on your age at the time you became disabled.

2. A duration of work test to show that you worked long enough under Social Security. Certain blind workers have to only meet the duration of work test.

Table 53.1 shows the rules for how much work you need for the recent work test, based on your age when your disability began. The following are the calendar quarters:
- **First quarter.** January 1 through March 31.
- **Second quarter.** April 1 through June 30.
- **Third quarter.** July 1 through September 30.
- **Fourth quarter.** October 1 through December 31.

Table 53.1. Rules on Determining Age for Each Calendar Quarter

If You Become Disabled…	Then You Generally Need:
In or before the quarter you turn age 24	1.5 years of work during the three-year period ending with the quarter your disability began.
In the quarter after you turn age 24 but before the quarter you turn age 31	Work during half the time for the period, beginning with the quarter after you turned 21 and ending with the quarter you became disabled. For example, if you become disabled in the quarter you turned age 27, then you would need three years of work out of the six-year period ending with the quarter you became disabled.
In the quarter you turn age 31 or later	Work during 5 years out of the 10-year period ending with the quarter your disability began.

Table 53.2 shows how many quarters of coverage you need to meet the duration of work test.

Table 53.2. Quarters of Coverage Necessary to Meet the Duration Requirement

If You Become Disabled…	Then You Generally Need:
Before age 28	1.5 years of work
Age 30	2 years
Age 34	3 years
Age 38	4 years

Disability Benefits for Multiple Sclerosis

Table 53.2. Continued

If You Become Disabled...	Then You Generally Need:
Age 42	5 years
Age 44	5.5 years
Age 46	6 years
Age 48	6.5 years
Age 50	7 years
Age 52	7.5 years
Age 54	8 years
Age 56	8.5 years
Age 58	9 years
Age 60	9.5 years

Note: You must have a minimum of six quarters of coverage to meet the duration requirement. This minimum requirement for six quarters of coverage is also applicable for those who have not yet attained age 22 and may apply for disability based on their own earnings.

HOW DO YOU APPLY FOR DISABILITY BENEFITS?

There are two ways that you can apply for disability benefits:
- Apply online at www.socialsecurity.gov.
- Call the U.S. Social Security Administration's (SSA) toll-free number, 800-772-1213, to make an appointment to file a disability claim at your local Social Security office or to set up an appointment for someone to take your claim over the telephone. The disability claims interview lasts about one hour. If you are deaf or hard of hearing, you may call SSA's toll-free teletypewriter (TTY) number, 800-325-0778, between 8 a.m. and 7 p.m. on business days. If you schedule an appointment, the SSA will send you a "Disability Starter Kit" to help you get ready for your disability claims interview. The Disability Starter Kit is also available online, through the SSA's website (www.ssa.gov/disability).

You have the right to representation by an attorney or other qualified person of your choice when you do business with Social Security.

WHEN SHOULD YOU APPLY AND WHAT INFORMATION DO YOU NEED?

You should apply for disability benefits as soon as you become disabled. Processing an application for disability benefits can take three to five months. To apply for disability benefits, you will need to complete an application for Social Security benefits. You can apply online at www.ssa.gov/applyfordisability. They may be able to process your application faster if you provide all the needed information.

The information needed includes:
- your Social Security number (SSN)
- your date and place of birth
- names, addresses, and phone numbers of the doctors, caseworkers, hospitals, and clinics that took care of you and the dates of your visits
- names and dosage of all the medicine you take
- medical records from your doctors, therapists, hospitals, clinics, and caseworkers that you already have in your possession
- laboratory and test results
- a summary of where you worked and the kind of work you did
- a copy of your most recent W-2 Form (Wage and Tax Statement) or, if you are self-employed, your federal tax returns for the past year

In addition to the basic application for disability benefits, you will also need to fill out other forms. One form collects information about your medical condition and how it affects your ability to work. Other forms give doctors, hospitals, and other health-care professionals who have treated you permission to send in information about your medical condition.

Do not delay applying for benefits if you cannot get all of this information together quickly; the SSA can help you get it.

Disability Benefits for Multiple Sclerosis

WHO DECIDES IF YOU HAVE A QUALIFYING DISABILITY?

The Social Security will review your application to make sure you meet some basic requirements for disability benefits. They will check whether you worked enough years to qualify and evaluate any current work activities. If you meet these requirements, the SSA will process your application and forward your case to the Disability Determination Services office in your state.

This state agency completes the initial disability determination decision for the SSA. Doctors and disability specialists in the state agency ask your doctors for information about your condition. They will consider all the facts in your case. They will use the medical evidence from your doctors, hospitals, clinics, or institutions where you have been treated and all other information. They will ask your doctors about:
- your medical condition(s)
- when your medical condition(s) began
- how your medical condition(s) limit your activities
- medical tests results
- what treatment you have received

They will also ask the doctors for information about your ability to do work-related activities, such as walking, sitting, lifting, carrying, and remembering instructions. Your doctors do not decide if you are disabled.

The state agency staff may need more medical information before they can decide if you are disabled. If your medical sources cannot provide the needed information, the state agency may ask you to go for a special examination. Social Security prefers this examination to be conducted by your own doctor, but, sometimes, the exam may have to be done by someone else. Social Security will pay for the exam and for some of the related travel costs.

HOW IS THE DECISION MADE?

The Social Security uses a five-step evaluation process, in a set order, to decide if you are disabled.

Are You Working?
If you are working, and your earnings average more than a certain amount each month, the SSA generally would not consider you to be disabled. The amount (referred to as "substantial gainful activity") changes each year.

If you are not working, or your monthly earnings average to the current amount or less, the state agency then looks at your medical condition at step two.

Is Your Medical Condition "Severe"?
For you to be considered to have a disability by Social Security's definition, your medical condition must significantly limit your ability to do basic work activities—such as lifting, standing, walking, sitting, and remembering—for at least 12 months. If your medical condition is not severe, the SSA will not consider you to be disabled. If your condition is severe, the Social Security proceeds to step three.

Does Your Medical Condition Meet or Medically Equal a Listing?
The Social Security has a listing of impairments (the listings) that describes medical conditions that are considered severe enough to prevent a person from doing any gainful activity, regardless of their age, education, or work experience. Within each listing, the SSA specifies the objective medical and other findings needed to satisfy the criteria of that listing. If your medical condition meets, or medically equals (meaning it is at least equal in severity and duration to), the criteria of a listing, the state agency will decide that you have a qualifying disability. If your medical condition does not meet or medically equal the criteria of a listing, the state agency goes on to step four.

Can You Do the Work You Did Before?
At this step, the Social Security decides if your medical condition(s) prevents you from performing any of your past work. If it does not, the SSA will decide that you do not have a qualifying disability. If it does, they will proceed to step five.

Can You Do Any Other Type of Work?
If you cannot do the work you did in the past, the SSA looks to see if there is other work you can do despite your medical condition(s). They consider your age, education, past work experience, and any skills you may have that could be used to do other work. If you cannot do other work, the SSA will decide that you are disabled. If you can do other work, they will decide that you do not have a qualifying disability.

WHAT HAPPENS WHEN YOUR CLAIM IS APPROVED
The Social Security will send a letter to tell you that your application is approved, the amount of your monthly benefit, and the effective date. Your monthly disability benefit is based on your average lifetime earnings. Your first Social Security disability benefits will be paid for the sixth full month after the date your disability began.

Here is an example: If the state agency decides your disability began on January 15, your first disability benefit will be paid for the month of July. The Social Security benefits are paid in the month following the month for which they are due, so you will receive your July benefit in August.

CAN YOUR FAMILY GET BENEFITS?
Certain members of your family may qualify for benefits based on your work. They include your:
- spouse, if he or she is 62 years of age or older
- spouse at any age, if he or she is caring for a child of yours who is younger than the age of 16 or disabled
- unmarried child, including an adopted child, or, in some cases, a stepchild or grandchild. The child must be younger than the age of 18 (or younger than 19 years of age if still in high school)
- unmarried child, 18 years of age or older, if he or she has a disability that started before the age of 22. The child's disability must also meet the definition of disability for adults

Note: *In some situations, a divorced spouse may qualify for benefits based on your earnings, if he or she was married to you for at least 10 years, is not currently married, and is at least 62 years of age. The money paid to a divorced spouse does not reduce your benefit or any benefits due to your current spouse or children.*

HOW DO OTHER PAYMENTS AFFECT YOUR BENEFITS?

If you are getting other government benefits (including those from a foreign country), the amount of your Social Security disability benefits may be affected.

WHAT DO YOU NEED TO TELL SOCIAL SECURITY?
If You Have an Outstanding Warrant for Your Arrest

You must tell the Social Security if you have an outstanding arrest warrant for any of the following felony offenses:
- flight to avoid prosecution or confinement
- escape from custody
- flight escape

You cannot receive regular disability benefits or any underpayments you may be due, for any month in which there is an outstanding arrest warrant for any of these felony offenses.

If You Are Convicted of a Crime

Tell Social Security right away if you are convicted of a crime. Regular disability benefits, or any underpayments that may be due, are not paid for the months a person is confined for a crime, but any family members who are eligible for benefits based on that person's work may continue to receive benefits.

Monthly benefits, or any underpayments that may be due, are usually not paid to someone who commits a crime and is confined to an institution by court order and at public expense. This applies if the person has been found:
- not guilty by reason of insanity or similar factors (such as mental disease, mental defect, or mental incompetence)
- incompetent to stand trial

Disability Benefits for Multiple Sclerosis

If you violate a condition of parole or probation, you must tell the SSA if you are violating a condition of your probation or parole, as imposed under federal or state law. You cannot receive regular disability benefits or any underpayment that may be due for any month in which you violate a condition of your probation or parole.

WHEN DO YOU GET MEDICARE?
You will get Medicare coverage automatically after you have received disability benefits for two years. You can find more information about the Medicare program, in the Medicare section of the SSA's website.

WHAT DO YOU NEED TO KNOW ABOUT WORKING?
After you start receiving Social Security disability benefits, you may want to try working again. Social Security has special rules, called "work incentives," that allow you to test your ability to work and still receive monthly Social Security disability benefits. You can also get help with education, rehabilitation, and training you may need to work.

If you do take a job or become self-employed, tell the SSA about it right away. They need to know when you start or stop work, and if there are any changes in your job duties, hours of work, or rate of pay. You can call them toll-free at 800-772-1213. If you are deaf or hard of hearing, you may call their teletypewriter (TTY) number, 800-325-0778.

For more information about helping you return to work, ask for the "Working While Disabled—How We Can Help" booklet. A guide to all of Social Security's employment supports can be found in SSA's "Red Book," which is a summary guide to employment support for individuals with disabilities under the SSDI and SSI programs.

THE TICKET TO WORK PROGRAM
Under the Ticket to Work program, the Social Security and SSI disability beneficiaries can get help with training and other services they need to go to work at no cost to them. Most disability

beneficiaries are eligible to participate in the Ticket to Work program and can select an approved provider of their choice who can offer the kind of services they need.

CONTACTING SOCIAL SECURITY

There are several ways to contact Social Security, including online, by phone, and in person. They are here to answer your questions and to serve you. For nearly 90 years, Social Security has helped secure today and tomorrow by providing benefits and financial protection for millions of people throughout their life's journey.

Visit Their Website

The most convenient way to conduct business with us is online at www.ssa.gov. You can accomplish a lot.
- Apply for Extra Help with Medicare prescription drug plan costs.
- Apply for most types of benefits.
- Start or complete your request for an original or replacement Social Security card.
- Find copies of our publications.
- Get answers to frequently asked questions.

When you create a personal my Social Security account, you can do even more.
- Review your Social Security statement.
- Verify your earnings.
- Get estimates of future benefits.
- Print a benefit verification letter.
- Change your direct deposit information.
- Request a replacement Medicare card.
- Get a replacement SSA-1099/1042S.

Access to your personal my Social Security account may be limited for users outside the United States.

Disability Benefits for Multiple Sclerosis

Call

If you cannot use our online services, the SSA can help you by phone when you call our National toll-free 800 number. The SSA provides free interpreter services upon request. They can call you at 800-772-1213—or at our teletypewriter (TTY) number, 800-325-0778, if you are deaf or hard of hearing—between 8:00 a.m. and 7:00 p.m., Monday through Friday. For quicker access to a representative, try calling early in the day (between 8 and 10 a.m. local time) or later in the day. The SSA is less busy later in the week (Wednesday to Friday) and later in the month. They also offer many automated telephone services, available 24 hours a day, so you may not need to speak with a representative. If you have documents they need to see, remember that they must be original or copies that are certified by the issuing agency.[1]

---

[1] "Disability Benefits," U.S. Social Security Administration (SSA), August 2022. Available online. URL: www.ssa.gov/pubs/EN-05-10029.pdf. Accessed March 1, 2024.

Chapter 54 | Building Support Networks with Multiple Sclerosis

Living with multiple sclerosis (MS) can be very challenging. It requires accepting those things you cannot change and adjusting to the "new normal" for you and your loved ones. This change in perspective helps shift your focus from the past to the present. Social workers are educated and trained to help you understand and accept the challenges of living with MS and assist you in finding ways to live your best life.

Social workers may work closely with you and your care partner. A social worker can work with your MS team and MS organizations to provide you with resources.

If you do not know who your social worker is, ask your primary care or MS provider to meet and talk with your social worker. Below are some of the roles of the MS social worker.

ROLE OF MULTIPLE SCLEROSIS SOCIAL WORKER

As a case manager on the MS team:
- Assess the needs of the MS people and family by completing a comprehensive psychosocial assessment and formulating a personalized plan.
- Identify community resources, implement referrals, and follow-up on the results.
- Partner with other professionals in mental health, primary care, and other service lines to provide

comprehensive management of resources, support systems, and services to people and care partners.

As an advocate on the MS team:
- Intercede and speak in defense of the people's well-being.
- Advocate for what the people desires in their care.
- Assist people in navigation of the health-care system and private sector.

As a counselor on the MS team:
- Provide supportive counseling to assist MS people's family members in coping with the effect of MS, changes in roles and identity, and disease progression.
- Provide psychotherapy in the form of crisis or long-term clinical intervention to assist MS people family members with mental health diagnoses and/or adjustment to life with MS.
- Provide coping strategies for managing emotions: sadness, anger, worry, and fear.

As a facilitator on the MS team:
- Seek opportunities to gather people together for peer support: MS support groups, telephone support groups, and/or caregiver support groups.
- Develop relationships with community organizations that support people with MS.
- Assess for and link care partners to appropriate U.S. Department of Veterans Affairs (VA) and community resources.

As an educator on the MS team:
- Inform the MS people/family members but also fellow team members on benefits, compensation programs, resources, support programs, and systems in place for people with MS and their care partners.

Building Support Networks with Multiple Sclerosis

- Provide education to MS people, families, and interdisciplinary team members on the psychosocial effect of illness and disease progression.
- Provide education on planning for care with the use of advanced directives and advance care planning.

As a negotiator on the MS team:
- Assist in resolving MS people and care partner conflicts and providing supportive counseling as appropriate.
- Assist in resolving systemic conflicts that effect the care of the MS people.[1]

---

[1] "Social Worker Support for Veterans and Families," U.S. Department of Veterans Affairs (VA), February 13, 2024. Available online. URL: www.va.gov/MS/RESOURCES/Emotional_Support_Services_for_Veterans_and_Families.asp. Accessed February 29, 2024.

Chapter 55 | Long-Term Care Options and Multiple Sclerosis

Sometimes an older person can no longer live safely or comfortably in their own home. Some people may be able to move in with family or friends. Others need more help than a family member or friend can provide. They might move to a residential (live-in) facility, such as a board and care home, a nursing home, an assisted living facility, or a continuing care retirement community.

A residential facility can provide some or all of the long-term care services an older person needs. Some facilities offer only housing and housekeeping, but many also provide personal care, social and recreational activities, meals, and medical services. Some facilities offer special programs for people with Alzheimer disease (AD) and other types of dementia.

BOARD AND CARE HOMES

These small private facilities, also called "residential care facilities" or "group homes," usually have 20 or fewer residents. Rooms may be private or shared. Residents receive personal care and meals, and staff are available around the clock. Nursing and medical care usually are not provided at the home.

In most cases, you must pay the costs of living at a board and care home. Medicare does not cover these costs. Medicaid may provide partial coverage, depending on the state and whether the person is eligible. If the older person has long-term care insurance, check their plan to see if it includes coverage for this type of facility.

ASSISTED LIVING

Assisted living is for people who need help with daily care but not as much help as a nursing home provides. Assisted living facilities range in size from as few as 25 residents to 100 or more. Typically, a few levels of care are offered, and residents pay more if they need extra services or special care.

Assisted living residents usually live in their own apartments or rooms and share common areas. They have access to many services, including up to three meals a day; assistance with personal care; help with medications, housekeeping, and laundry; 24-hour supervision, security, and on-site staff; and social and recreational activities. Some assisted living facilities are part of a larger organization that also offers other levels of care. For example, continuing care retirement communities (CCRCs) may also offer independent living and skilled nursing care. Exact arrangements vary by facility and by state.

Most people pay the full costs of assisted living themselves. This option tends to be more expensive than living independently but less expensive than a nursing home. Medicare does not pay for assisted living. Medicaid may provide coverage for some aspects of assisted living, depending on the state and whether the person is eligible. This care option is partially covered by some long-term care insurance policies.

NURSING HOMES

Nursing homes, also called "skilled nursing facilities," provide a wide range of health and personal care services. Their services focus more on medical care than most assisted living facilities or board and care homes. Services offered in a nursing home typically include nursing care, 24-hour supervision, three meals a day, and assistance with everyday activities. Rehabilitation services, such as physical, occupational, and speech therapy, are also available.

In many cases, people must pay for nursing home care themselves. Medicare generally does not cover long-term stays in a nursing home, but it may pay for some related costs, such as doctor services and medical supplies. Medicaid may also cover some of the costs of nursing homes for people who are eligible based on income and personal resources. If the older person has long-term care insurance, the policy may include some coverage for nursing home care.

CONTINUING CARE RETIREMENT COMMUNITIES

Continuing care retirement communities, also called "life care communities," offer different levels of service in one location. Many of them offer independent housing (in houses or apartments), assisted living, and skilled nursing care, all on one campus. Healthcare services and recreation programs are also provided.

In a CCRC, where you live depends on the level of service you need. People who can no longer live independently move to the assisted living facility or sometimes receive home care in their independent living unit. If necessary, they can enter the CCRC's nursing home.

Most CCRCs charge a one-time entrance fee, which may be relatively expensive, and a monthly fee after that. People must pay most of these costs themselves. Medicare, Medicaid, and long-term care insurance may cover some services, depending on the level of care provided.[1]

---

[1] National Institute on Aging (NIA), "Long-Term Care Facilities: Assisted Living, Nursing Homes, and Other Residential Care," National Institutes of Health (NIH), October 12, 2023. Available online. URL: www.nia.nih.gov/health/assisted-living-and-nursing-homes/long-term-care-facilities-assisted-living-nursing-homes. Accessed February 29, 2024.

Chapter 56 | Guide to Disability Rights Laws

THE AMERICANS WITH DISABILITIES ACT
The Americans with Disabilities Act (ADA) prohibits discrimination on the basis of disability in employment, state and local government, public accommodations, commercial facilities, transportation, and telecommunications. It also applies to the United States Congress.

To be protected by the ADA, one must have a disability or have a relationship or association with an individual with a disability. An individual with a disability is defined by the ADA as a person who has a physical or mental impairment that substantially limits one or more major life activities, a person who has a history or record of such an impairment, or a person who is perceived by others as having such an impairment. The ADA does not specifically name all of the impairments that are covered.

ADA Title I: Employment
Title I requires employers with 15 or more employees to provide qualified individuals with disabilities an equal opportunity to benefit from the full range of employment-related opportunities available to others. For example, it prohibits discrimination in recruitment, hiring, promotions, training, pay, social activities, and other privileges of employment. It restricts questions that can be asked about an applicant's disability before a job offer is made, and it requires that employers make reasonable accommodation to the known physical or mental limitations of otherwise qualified individuals with disabilities, unless it results in undue hardship.

Religious entities with 15 or more employees are covered under title I.

Title I complaints must be filed with the U. S. Equal Employment Opportunity Commission (EEOC) within 180 days of the date of discrimination, or 300 days if the charge is filed with a designated state or local fair employment practice agency. Individuals may file a lawsuit in federal court only after they receive a "right-to-sue" letter from the EEOC.

Charges of employment discrimination on the basis of disability may be filed at any EEOC field office. Field offices are located in 50 cities throughout the United States and are listed in most telephone directories under "U.S. Government."

ADA Title II: State and Local Government Activities

Title II covers all activities of state and local governments regardless of the government entity's size or receipt of federal funding. Title II requires that state and local governments give people with disabilities an equal opportunity to benefit from all of their programs, services, and activities (e.g., public education, employment, transportation, recreation, health care, social services, courts, voting, and town meetings).

State and local governments are required to follow specific architectural standards in the new construction and alteration of their buildings. They also must relocate programs or otherwise provide access in inaccessible older buildings and communicate effectively with people who have hearing, vision, or speech disabilities. Public entities are not required to take actions that would result in undue financial and administrative burdens. They are required to make reasonable modifications to policies, practices, and procedures where necessary to avoid discrimination, unless they can demonstrate that doing so would fundamentally alter the nature of the service, program, or activity being provided.

Complaints of title II violations may be filed with the Department of Justice (DOJ) within 180 days of the date of discrimination. In certain situations, cases may be referred to a mediation program sponsored by the DOJ. The DOJ may bring a lawsuit where it has investigated a matter and has been unable to resolve violations.

Guide to Disability Rights Laws

Title II may also be enforced through private lawsuits in federal court. It is not necessary to file a complaint with the DOJ or any other federal agency or to receive a "right-to-sue" letter, before going to court.

ADA Title II: Public Transportation

The transportation provisions of title II cover public transportation services, such as city buses and public rail transit (e.g., subways, commuter rails, and Amtrak). Public transportation authorities may not discriminate against people with disabilities in the provision of their services. They must comply with requirements for accessibility in newly purchased vehicles, make good faith efforts to purchase or lease accessible used buses, remanufacture buses in an accessible manner and, unless it would result in an undue burden, provide paratransit where they operate fixed-route bus or rail systems. Paratransit is a service where individuals who are unable to use the regular transit system independently (because of a physical or mental impairment) are picked up and dropped off at their destinations.

ADA Title III: Public Accommodations

Title III covers businesses and nonprofit service providers that are public accommodations, privately operated entities offering certain types of courses and examinations, privately operated transportation, and commercial facilities. Public accommodations are private entities who own, lease, lease to, or operate facilities such as restaurants, retail stores, hotels, movie theaters, private schools, convention centers, doctors' offices, homeless shelters, transportation depots, zoos, funeral homes, day care centers, and recreation facilities including sports stadiums and fitness clubs. Transportation services provided by private entities are also covered by title III.

Public accommodations must comply with basic nondiscrimination requirements that prohibit exclusion, segregation, and unequal treatment. They also must comply with specific requirements related to architectural standards for new and altered buildings; reasonable modifications to policies, practices, and procedures; effective communication with people with hearing, vision, or speech disabilities; and other access requirements. Additionally, public accommodations must remove barriers in existing buildings where it is easy to do so without much difficulty or expense, given the public accommodation's resources.

Courses and examinations related to professional, educational, or trade-related applications, licensing, certifications, or credentialing must be provided in a place and manner accessible to people with disabilities, or alternative accessible arrangements must be offered.

Commercial facilities, such as factories and warehouses, must comply with the ADA's architectural standards for new construction and alterations.

Complaints of title III violations may be filed with the DOJ. In certain situations, cases may be referred to a mediation program sponsored by the DOJ. The DOJ is authorized to bring a lawsuit where there is a pattern or practice of discrimination in violation of title III or where an act of discrimination raises an issue of general public importance. Title III may also be enforced through private lawsuits.

ADA Title IV: Telecommunications Relay Services

Title IV addresses telephone and television access for people with hearing and speech disabilities. It requires common carriers (telephone companies) to establish interstate and intrastate telecommunications relay services (TRS) 24 hours a day, 7 days a week. TRS enables callers with hearing and speech disabilities who use teletypewriters (TTYs; also known as "telecommunications device for the deaf" (TDDs)), and callers who use voice telephones to communicate with each other through a third-party communications assistant. The Federal Communications Commission (FCC) has set minimum standards for TRS services. Title IV also requires closed captioning of federally funded public service announcements.

TELECOMMUNICATIONS ACT

Section 255 and Section 251(a)(2) of the Communications Act of 1934, as amended by the Telecommunications Act of 1996, require manufacturers of telecommunications equipment and providers of telecommunications services to ensure that such equipment and services are accessible to and usable by persons with disabilities, if readily achievable. These amendments ensure that people with disabilities will have access to a broad range of products and services, such as telephones, cell phones, pagers, call-waiting, and operator services, that were often inaccessible to many users with disabilities.

FAIR HOUSING ACT

The Fair Housing Act, as amended in 1988, prohibits housing discrimination on the basis of race, color, religion, sex, disability, familial status, and national origin. Its coverage includes private housing, housing that receives federal financial assistance, and state and local government housing. It is unlawful to discriminate in any aspect of selling or renting housing or to deny a dwelling to a buyer or renter because of the disability of that individual, an individual associated with the buyer or renter, or an individual who intends to live in the residence. Other covered activities include, for example, financing, zoning practices, new construction design, and advertising.

The Fair Housing Act requires owners of housing facilities to make reasonable exceptions in their policies and operations to afford people with disabilities equal housing opportunities. For example, a landlord with a "no pets" policy may be required to grant an exception to this rule and allow an individual who is blind to keep a guide dog in the residence. The Fair Housing Act also requires landlords to allow tenants with disabilities to make reasonable access-related modifications to their private living space, as well as to common use spaces. (The landlord is not required to pay for the changes.) The Fair Housing Act further requires that new multifamily housing with four or more units be designed and built to allow access for persons with disabilities. This includes accessible common use areas, doors that are wide enough for wheelchairs, kitchens, and bathrooms that allow a person using a wheelchair to maneuver and other adaptable features within the units.

Additionally, the DOJ can file cases involving a pattern or practice of discrimination. The Fair Housing Act may also be enforced through private lawsuits.

AIR CARRIER ACCESS ACT

The Air Carrier Access Act (ACAA) prohibits discrimination in air transportation by domestic and foreign air carriers against qualified individuals with physical or mental impairments. It applies only to air carriers that provide regularly scheduled services for hire to the public. Requirements address a wide range of issues, including boarding assistance and certain accessibility features in newly built aircraft and new or altered airport facilities. People may enforce rights under the ACAA by filing a complaint with the U.S. Department of Transportation (DOT) or by bringing a lawsuit in federal court.

VOTING ACCESSIBILITY FOR THE ELDERLY AND HANDICAPPED ACT

The Voting Accessibility for the Elderly and Handicapped Act (VAEHA) of 1984 generally requires polling places across the United States to be physically accessible to people with disabilities for federal elections. Where no accessible location is available to serve as a polling place, a political subdivision must provide an alternate means of casting a ballot on the day of the election. This law also requires states to make available registration and voting aids for disabled and elderly voters, including information by TTYs or similar devices.

NATIONAL VOTER REGISTRATION ACT

The National Voter Registration Act (NVRA) of 1993, also known as the "Motor Voter Act," makes it easier for all Americans to exercise their fundamental right to vote. One of the basic purposes of the NVRA is to increase the historically low registration rates of minorities and persons with disabilities that have resulted from discrimination. The NVRA requires all offices of state-funded programs that are primarily engaged in providing services to persons with disabilities to provide all program applicants with voter registration forms, to assist them in completing the forms, and to transmit completed forms to the appropriate state official.

CIVIL RIGHTS OF INSTITUTIONALIZED PERSONS ACT

The Civil Rights of Institutionalized Persons Act (CRIPA) authorizes the U.S. Attorney General to investigate conditions of confinement at state and local government institutions such as prisons, jails, pretrial detention centers, juvenile correctional facilities, publicly operated nursing homes, and institutions for people with psychiatric or developmental disabilities. Its purpose is to allow the Attorney General to uncover and correct widespread deficiencies that seriously jeopardize the health and safety of residents of institutions. The Attorney General does not have authority under the CRIPA to investigate isolated incidents or to represent individual institutionalized persons.

The Attorney General may initiate civil lawsuits where there is reasonable cause to believe that conditions are "egregious or flagrant," that they are subjecting residents to "grievous harm," and that they are part of a "pattern or practice" of resistance to residents' full enjoyment of constitutional or federal rights, including title II of the ADA and Section 504 of the Rehabilitation Act.

INDIVIDUALS WITH DISABILITIES EDUCATION ACT

The Individuals with Disabilities Education Act (IDEA; formerly called "P.L. 94-142" or the "Education for All Handicapped Children Act of 1975") requires public schools to make available to all eligible children with disabilities a free appropriate public education in the least restrictive environment appropriate to their individual needs.

The IDEA requires public school systems to develop appropriate Individualized Education Programs (IEPs) for each child. The specific special education and related services outlined in each IEP reflect the individualized needs of each student.

The IDEA also mandates that particular procedures be followed in the development of the IEP. Each student's IEP must be developed by a team of knowledgeable persons and must be at least reviewed annually. The team includes the child's teacher; the parents, subject to certain limited exceptions; the child, if determined appropriate; an agency representative who is qualified to provide or supervise the provision of special education; and other individuals at the parents' or agency's discretion.

If parents disagree with the proposed IEP, they can request a due process hearing and a review from the state educational agency if applicable in that state. They also can appeal the State agency's decision to state or federal court.

REHABILITATION ACT

The Rehabilitation Act prohibits discrimination on the basis of disability in programs conducted by federal agencies, in programs receiving federal financial assistance, in federal employment, and in the employment practices of federal contractors. The standards for determining employment discrimination under the Rehabilitation Act are the same as those used in title I of the ADA.

Section 501

Section 501 requires affirmative action and nondiscrimination in employment by federal agencies of the executive branch. To obtain more information or to file a complaint, employees should contact their agency's EEOC.

Section 503

Section 503 requires affirmative action and prohibits employment discrimination by federal government contractors and subcontractors with contracts of more than $10,000.

Section 504

Section 504 states that "no qualified individual with a disability in the United States shall be excluded from, denied the benefits of, or be subjected to discrimination under" any program or activity that either receives federal financial assistance or is conducted by any Executive agency or the United States Postal Service (USPS).

Each federal agency has its own set of Section 504 regulations that apply to its own programs. Agencies that provide federal financial assistance also have Section 504 regulations covering entities that receive federal aid. Requirements common to these regulations include reasonable accommodation for employees with disabilities; program accessibility; effective communication with people who have hearing or vision disabilities; and accessible new construction and alterations. Each agency is responsible for enforcing its own regulations. Section 504 may also be enforced through private lawsuits. It is not necessary to file a complaint with a federal agency or to receive a "right-to-sue" letter before going to court.

Section 508

Section 508 establishes requirements for electronic and information technology developed, maintained, procured, or used by the federal government. Section 508 requires federal electronic and information technology to be accessible to people with disabilities, including employees and members of the public.

An accessible information technology system is one that can be operated in a variety of ways and does not rely on a single sense or ability of the user. For example, a system that provides output only in visual format may not be accessible to people with visual impairments and a system that provides output only in audio format may not be accessible to people who are deaf or hard of hearing. Some individuals with disabilities may need accessibility-related software or peripheral devices in order to use systems that comply with Section 508.

ARCHITECTURAL BARRIERS ACT

The Architectural Barriers Act (ABA) requires that buildings and facilities that are designed, constructed, or altered with federal funds, or leased by a federal agency, comply with federal standards for physical accessibility. ABA requirements are limited to architectural standards in new and altered buildings and in newly leased facilities. They do not address the activities conducted in those buildings and facilities. Facilities of the USPS are covered by the ABA.[1]

---

[1] ADA.gov, "Guide to Disability Rights Laws," U.S. Department of Justice (DOJ), February 28, 2020. Available online. URL: www.ada.gov/resources/disability-rights-guide. Accessed February 29, 2024.

Chapter 57 | Guardianship for People with Disability

According to the National Guardianship Association (NGA), Inc., "Guardianship, also referred to as 'conservatorship,' is a legal process, utilized when a person can no longer make or communicate safe or sound decisions about his/her person and/or property or has become susceptible to fraud or undue influence. Because establishing a guardianship may remove considerable rights from an individual, it should only be considered after alternatives to guardianship have proven ineffective or are unavailable."

Before evaluating guardianship or making recommendations for how to improve it, it is important to define and ensure a basic understanding of what guardianship is. Although the previous quote may seem like a reasonable definition, it contains value judgments—which are worthy of consideration—such as what constitutes "safe or sound decisions," who gets to make that determination for an individual, and how an individual's safety should balance against his or her right to experience the dignity of risk.

Despite the oft-cited proposition that all people have certain inalienable rights, once someone is declared incapacitated and is appointed a guardian, many of their rights are taken away, and their ability to make decisions in a wide variety of areas is given to another person.

Therefore, although guardianship is largely a creature of state law, it nonetheless raises fundamental questions concerning federal civil rights and constitutional due process. An adult usually becomes subject to guardianship when the court finds that:
- the individual is incapable of making all or some of their own financial or personal decisions

- it is necessary to appoint a guardian to make those choices on their behalf

RIGHTS AT RISK IN GUARDIANSHIPS

Guardianships are typically separated into two categories, guardianships of the person and guardianships of the property (also sometimes referred to as "conservatorship"). When the guardian controls decisions regarding both person and property, the guardianship is called "plenary." However, there are really three types of rights that are at issue in guardianships:
- rights that can be taken from an individual but not given to another individual
- rights that can be taken from a person and exercised by someone else on their behalf
- rights that a guardian needs a court order to exercise on the individual's behalf

A person who is determined incapacitated generally can have the following rights removed, but these rights cannot be exercised by someone else. These include the right to:
- marry
- vote
- drive
- seek or retain employment

Still, other rights can be removed and transferred to a guardian who can exercise these rights on behalf of the individual, such as the right to:
- contract
- sue and defend lawsuits
- apply for government benefits
- manage money or property
- decide where to live
- consent to medical treatment
- decide with whom to associate or be friends

In many states, there are also some rights that a guardian can exercise on behalf of the individual subject to guardianship, but

only after the court has issued a specific order allowing the action, such as:
- committing the person to a facility or institution
- consenting to biomedical or behavioral experiments
- filing for divorce
- consenting to the termination of parental rights
- consenting to sterilization or abortion

A WORD ON LANGUAGE

When a petition is filed with the court that alleges that the individual is incapacitated, the individual is often referred to as the "alleged incapacitated person" (AIP). If the court finds that the person does lack capacity and appoints a guardian to manage some or all of their affairs, the individual is often referred to as the "ward."

In this report, the term AIP will be used, but because the term "ward" is viewed by many as stigmatizing and inappropriate, whenever possible, consistent with National Council on Disability's (NCD) longstanding commitment of avoiding stigmatizing language, individuals for whom a guardian has been appointed as an individual subject to guardianship will be referred to. This is also consistent with the Uniform Guardianship, Conservatorship, and Other Protective Arrangements Act (UGCOPAA), which is the latest iteration of the uniform guardianship statute that has been approved by the Uniform Law Commission (ULC). However, it should be noted that the term "ward" will appear when it appears in a direct quote.

PROCESS OF OBTAINING GUARDIANSHIP

Guardianship petitions may be filed in a wide variety of situations, such as by parents when a child with an intellectual disability reaches 18 years of age, by a son or daughter when a parent begins to show signs of dementia severe enough that there is concern for their safety, for a person with a severe disability due to sudden trauma, or when there is concern that a bad actor is exercising undue influence over a person with a disability in order to exploit the individual in some way. There are also times when guardianship is filed for less altruistic reasons, such as to gain access to the person's assets or public benefits or to exploit the individual. Whether the guardianship is over person, property, or both, or whether it is limited or plenary may be determined, at least in part, by the circumstances that give rise to the perceived need for guardianship. Due to our federalist system of government, guardianship is a creature of state, rather than federal law, and all 50 states and the District of Columbia have revised their statutes regarding guardianship numerous times.

However, it is not clear that, in statute or in practice, guardianship law has been able to keep pace with the nation's changing understanding of disability, autonomy, and due process. Although the process is different in every state, making it difficult to provide a singular description of the guardianship process, there are certain generalities that are helpful to discuss before examination of whether or not guardianship is working for people with disabilities, their families, and communities. The following steps are generalities that may or may not align with the laws in a given state, so it is important for interested individuals to consult their state's laws for more accurate, detailed information.

General Steps to Guardianship
- filing the petitions
- notice that a guardianship petition has been filed
- appointment of an attorney to represent the AIP
- capacity evaluation
- hearing
- letters of guardianship
- guardianship plan and initial reports

GUARDIANSHIP AS A DISABILITY POLICY ISSUE
Guardianship is often overlooked, and, when it becomes part of the national policy conversation, it is often viewed as an issue affecting older Americans and not thought of as an important disability issue. However, guardianship must be understood as a disability policy issue worthy of examination, reflection, and reform. After

Guardianship for People with Disability

all, an adult becomes subject to guardianship only if a court has determined that he or she cannot manage property or meet essential requirements for health and safety.

In order to fully understand guardianship as a disability issue, people need to come from a common understanding of it within the context of the evolution of disability policy, particularly as it relates to issues of liberty, autonomy, and self-determination.[1]

---

[1] "Beyond Guardianship: Toward Alternatives That Promote Greater Self-Determination," National Council on Disability (NCD), March 22, 2018. Available online. URL: www.govinfo.gov/content/pkg/GOVPUB-Y3_D63_3-PURL-gpo90585/pdf/GOVPUB-Y3_D63_3-PURL-gpo90585.pdf. Accessed March 1, 2024.

Chapter 58 | Advance Care Planning

WHAT IS ADVANCE CARE PLANNING?
Advance care planning involves discussing and preparing for future decisions about your medical care if you become seriously ill or unable to communicate your wishes. Having meaningful conversations with your loved ones is the most important part of advance care planning. Many people also choose to put their preferences in writing by completing legal documents called "advance directives."

WHAT ARE ADVANCE DIRECTIVES?
Advance directives are legal documents that provide instructions for medical care and only go into effect if you cannot communicate your own wishes.

The two most common advance directives for health care are the living will and the durable power of attorney for health care.
- **Living will.** A living will is a legal document that tells doctors how you want to be treated if you cannot make your own decisions about emergency treatment. In a living will, you can say which common medical treatments or care you would want, which ones you would want to avoid, and under which conditions each of your choices applies.
- **Durable power of attorney for health care.** A durable power of attorney for health care is a legal document that names your health-care proxy, a person who can make health-care decisions for you if you are unable to communicate these yourself. Your proxy, also known as a

"representative," "surrogate," or "agent," should be familiar with your values and wishes. A proxy can be chosen in addition to or instead of a living will. Having a health-care proxy helps you plan for situations that cannot be foreseen, such as a serious car accident or stroke.

Think of your advance directives as living documents that you review at least once each year and update if a major life event occurs, such as retirement, moving out of state, or a significant change in your health.[1]

TYPES OF ADVANCE DIRECTIVES

A health-care proxy is a document that names someone you trust to make health decisions if you cannot. This is also called a "durable power of attorney."

A living will tells which treatment you want if your life is threatened, including dialysis and breathing machines; resuscitation; tube feeding; and organ or tissue donation after you die.

HOW TO GET ADVANCE DIRECTIVES

Get an advance directive from any of these:
- your health-care provider
- your attorney
- your local Area Agency on Aging
- your state health department[2]

WHO NEEDS AN ADVANCE CARE PLAN?

Advance care planning is not just for people who are very old or ill. At any age, a medical crisis could leave you unable to communicate

---

[1] National Institute on Aging (NIA), "Advance Care Planning: Advance Directives for Health Care," National Institutes of Health (NIH), October 31, 2022. Available online. URL: www.nia.nih.gov/health/advance-care-planning/advance-care-planning-advance-directives-health-care#decisions. Accessed March 1, 2024.

[2] "Advance Directives & Long-Term Care," Centers for Medicare & Medicaid Services (CMS), August 17, 2012. Available online. URL: www.medicare.gov/manage-your-health/advance-directives-long-term-care. Accessed March 1, 2024.

Advance Care Planning

your own health-care decisions. Planning now for your future health care can help ensure you get the medical care you want and that someone you trust will be there to make decisions for you.

WHAT HAPPENS IF YOU DO NOT HAVE AN ADVANCE DIRECTIVE?

If you do not have an advance directive and you are unable to make decisions on your own, the state laws where you live will determine who may make medical decisions on your behalf. This is typically your spouse, your parents if they are available, or your children if they are adults. If you are unmarried and have not named your partner as your proxy, it is possible they could be excluded from decision-making. If you have no family members, some states allow a close friend who is familiar with your values to help. Or they may assign a physician to represent your best interests. To find out the laws in your state, contact your state legal aid office or state bar association.

WILL AN ADVANCE DIRECTIVE GUARANTEE YOUR WISHES ARE FOLLOWED?

An advance directive is legally recognized but not legally binding. This means that your health-care provider and proxy will do their best to respect your advance directives, but there may be circumstances in which they cannot follow your wishes exactly. For example, you may be in a complex medical situation where it is unclear what you would want. This is another key reason why having conversations about your preferences is so important. Talking with your loved ones ahead of time may help them better navigate unanticipated issues.

There is the possibility that a health-care provider refuses to follow your advance directives. This might happen if the decision goes against:

- the health-care provider's conscience
- the health-care institution's policy
- accepted health-care standards

In these situations, the health-care provider must inform your health-care proxy immediately and consider transferring your care to another provider.

OTHER ADVANCE CARE PLANNING FORMS AND ORDERS

You might want to prepare documents to express your wishes about a single medical issue or something else not already covered in your advance directives, such as an emergency. For these types of situations, you can talk with a doctor about establishing the following orders:

- **Do not resuscitate (DNR) order.** A DNR becomes part of your medical chart to inform medical staff in a hospital or nursing facility that you do not want cardiopulmonary resuscitation (CPR) or other CPR measures to be attempted if your heartbeat and breathing stop. Sometimes this document is referred to as a "do not attempt resuscitation" (DNAR) order or an "allow natural death" (AND) order. Even though a living will states that CPR is not wanted, it is helpful to have a DNR order as part of your medical file if you go to a hospital. Posting a DNR next to your hospital bed might avoid confusion in an emergency. Without a DNR order, medical staff will attempt every effort to restore your breathing and the normal rhythm of your heart.
- **Do not intubate (DNI) order.** A similar document, a DNI informs medical staff in a hospital or nursing facility that you do not want to be on a ventilator.
- **Do not hospitalize (DNH) order.** A DNH indicates to long-term care providers, such as nursing home staff, that you prefer not to be sent to a hospital for treatment at the end of life.
- **Out-of-hospital DNR order.** An out-of-hospital DNR alerts emergency medical personnel to your wishes regarding measures to restore your heartbeat or breathing if you are not in a hospital.
- **Physician orders for life-sustaining treatment (POLST) and medical orders for life-sustaining treatment (MOLST) forms.** These forms provide guidance about your medical care that health-care professionals can act on immediately in an emergency.

Advance Care Planning

They serve as a medical order in addition to your advance directive. Typically, you create a POLST or MOLST when you are near the end-of-life or critically ill and understand the specific decisions that might need to be made on your behalf. These forms may also be called "portable medical orders" or "physician orders for scope of treatment" (POST). Check with your state department of health to find out if these forms are available where you live.

You may also want to document your wishes about organ and tissue donation and brain donation. As well, learning about care options such as palliative care and hospice care can help you plan ahead.

HOW CAN YOU GET STARTED WITH ADVANCE CARE PLANNING?

To get started with advance care planning, consider the following steps:
- **Reflect on your values and wishes.** This can help you think through what matters most at the end of life and guide your decisions about future care and medical treatment.
- **Talk with your doctor about advance directives.** Advance care planning is covered by Medicare as part of your annual wellness visit. If you have private health insurance, check with your insurance provider. Talking to a health-care provider can help you learn about your current health and the kinds of decisions that are likely to come up. For example, you might ask about the decisions you may face if your high blood pressure leads to a stroke.
- **Choose someone you trust to make medical decisions for you.** Whether it is a family member, a loved one, or your lawyer, it is important to choose someone you trust as your health-care proxy. Once you have decided, discuss your values and preferences with them. If you are not ready to discuss specific treatments or care decisions yet, try talking about your general preferences. You can also try

other ways to share your wishes, such as writing a letter or watching a video on the topic together.
- **Complete your advance directive forms.** To make your care and treatment decisions official, you can complete a living will. Similarly, once you decide on your health-care proxy, you can make it official by completing a durable power of attorney for health care.
- **Share your forms with your health-care proxy, doctors, and loved ones.** After you have completed your advance directives, make copies and store them in a safe place. Give copies to your health-care proxy, health-care providers, and lawyer. Some states have registries that can store your advance directive for quick access by health-care providers and your proxy.
- **Keep the conversation going.** Continue to talk about your wishes and update your forms at least once each year or after major life changes. If you update your forms, file and keep your previous versions. Note the date the older copy was replaced by a new one. If you use a registry, make sure the latest version is on record.

Everyone approaches the process differently. Remember to be flexible and take it one step at a time. Start small. For example, try simply talking with your loved ones about what you appreciate and enjoy most about life. Your values, treatment preferences, and even the people you involve in your plan may change over time. The most important part is to start the conversation.

HOW TO FIND ADVANCE DIRECTIVE FORMS

You can establish your advance directives for little or no cost. Many states have their own forms that you can access and complete for free. Here are some ways you might find free advance directive forms in your state:
- Contact your State Attorney General's Office.
- Contact your local Area Agency on Aging. You can find your area agency phone number by visiting the Eldercare Locator or by calling 800-677-1116.

Advance Care Planning

- Download your state's form online from one of these national organizations: American Association of Retired Persons (AARP), American Bar Association (ABA), or National Hospice and Palliative Care Organization (NHPCO).
- If you are a veteran, contact your local U.S. Department of Veterans Affairs (VA) office. The VA offers an advance directive specifically for veterans.

Some people spend a lot of time in more than one state. If that is your situation, consider preparing advance directives using the form for each state and keep a copy in each place, too.

There are also organizations that enable you to create, download, and print your forms online, but they may charge fees. Before you pay, remember there are several ways to get your forms for free. Some free online resources include the following:

- **PREPARE for Your Care**. An interactive online program that was funded in part by National Institute on Aging (NIA).
- **The Conversation Project**. The Conversation Project is a public engagement initiative led by the Institute for Health Care Improvement.

If you use forms from a website, check to make sure they are legally recognized in your state. You should also make sure the website is secure and will protect your personal information.

Some people also choose to carry a card in their wallet, indicating they have an advance directive and where it is kept.[3]

---

[3] See footnote [1].

Part 6 | **Additional Help and Information**

Chapter 59 | Glossary of Terms Related to Multiple Sclerosis

adverse effect: An unexpected medical problem, also called an "adverse event" that happens during treatment with a drug or other therapy.

antigen: Any substance that causes the body to make an immune response against that substance.

aspiration: The accidental breathing in of food or fluid into the lungs.

assistive devices: Tools that enable individuals with disabilities to perform essential job functions (e.g., telephone headsets, adapted computer keyboards, and enhanced computer monitors).

atrophy: The process of wasting away or deteriorating in cells, tissues, and organs.

autoimmune disease: A condition in which the body recognizes its own tissues as foreign and directs an immune response against them.

autoimmune disorder: A condition in which the body's immune system attacks and destroys healthy body tissue by mistake.

axon: A nerve fiber in the peripheral nervous system that conducts impulses away from the cell body.

baclofen: A drug that relaxes muscles by blocking certain nerve receptors in the spinal cord.

blood-brain barrier (BBB): A layer of tightly packed cells that control the movement of substances between the blood and the fluid that surrounds the brain's neurons.

This glossary contains terms excerpted from documents produced by several sources deemed reliable.

calcium: A mineral that is an essential nutrient for bone health and for the proper functioning of the heart, muscles, and nerves.

central nervous system (CNS): The part of the nervous system that is made up of the brain and spinal cord. The CNS serves as the main processing center for the entire nervous system and coordinates all body functions.

cerebral: A term used to describe the principal part of the brain.

cerebrospinal fluid (CSF): The fluid that surrounds and fills the brain and spinal cord and protects the brain, provides nourishment for cells, and removes waste.

chronic disease: A disease that is permanent, leaves residual disability, is caused by nonreversible pathological alteration, requires special training of the patient for rehabilitation, or may be expected to require a long period of supervision, observation, or care.

chronic pain: Pain that can range from mild to severe and persists or progresses over a long period of time.

cognitive impairment: Problems with a person's ability to think, learn, remember, use judgment, and make decisions.

coma: A long, deep state of unconsciousness.

computed tomography (CT): A procedure for taking x-ray images from many different angles and then assembling them into a cross-section of the body.

constipation: A decrease in frequency of stools or bowel movements with hardening of the stool.

contracture: The shortening or tightening of the muscles or tendons around a person's joints.

cytokines: A type of protein that is made by certain immune and nonimmune cells and has an effect on the immune system.

dendrites: Part of the neuron that receives signals from other nerve cells.

diet: What a person eats and drinks.

dysphagia: Difficulty in swallowing and may even experience pain while swallowing (odynophagia).

dystonia: Involuntary muscle contractions or flexing that can cause slow repetitive movements or abnormal postures that can be painful.

Glossary of Terms Related to Multiple Sclerosis

enzymes: Proteins that help speed up chemical reactions in the body (called "metabolism").

epilepsy: Chronic brain disorder in which groups of nerve cells, or neurons, in the brain sometimes send the wrong signals and cause seizures.

exercise: A type of physical activity that involves planned, structured, and repetitive bodily movement done to maintain or improve one or more components of physical fitness.

fatigue: An extreme sense of tiredness and lack of energy that can interfere with a person's usual daily activities.

fetus: A developing unborn offspring in the uterus (womb).

Guillain-Barré syndrome (GBS): A rare neurological disorder in which a person's immune system mistakenly attacks part of their peripheral nervous system—the network of nerves that carries signals from the brain and spinal cord to the rest of the body.

immune system: The immune system is the body's way of protecting itself from infection and disease; it fights everything from cold and flu viruses to serious conditions such as cancer.

inflammation: A condition in which tissues, organs, or other parts of the body become swollen, hot, or painful.

lesion: An area of abnormal tissue that may be benign (not cancer) or malignant (cancer).

magnetic resonance imaging (MRI): A noninvasive procedure that uses magnetic fields and radio waves to produce three-dimensional computerized images of areas inside the body.

multiple sclerosis (MS): A disorder of the brain and spinal cord that causes decreased nerve function associated with the formation of scars on the covering of nerve cells.

myelin: A fatty molecule that provides insulation for the axon and helps nerve signals travel faster and farther.

neuroimaging: The process of determining the structure or function of the brain through various imaging techniques.

neuromyelitis optica (NMO): An autoimmune disease of the CNS that mainly affects the optic nerves and spinal cord.

neuron: Also called "nerve cells," neurons are the primary communication cells that send messages from the brain all over the body.

neurotransmitter: A chemical produced by neurons that carry messages from one nerve cell to another.

nutrition: The taking in and use of food and other nourishing material by the body.

oligodendrocyte: A cell that forms the myelin sheath (a layer that covers and protects nerve cells) in the brain and spinal cord.

paralysis: An inability to move parts of the body accompanied by a loss of sensation.

paresthesia: A burning, itching, tingling, or prickling sensation that is usually felt in the hands, arms, legs, or feet.

peripheral nervous system (PNS): Nerves that branch out from the brain and spinal cord to reach all other parts of the body.

physical activity: Any bodily movement that is produced by the contraction of skeletal muscle and that substantially increases energy expenditure.

plasmapheresis: A procedure in which blood is removed, immune system cells and antibodies are taken out, and the blood is separated into plasma and blood cells.

pregnancy: The condition between conception (fertilization of an egg by a sperm) and birth, during which the fertilized egg develops in the uterus.

Schilder disease: An extremely rare disease that involves the breakdown of the protective coating (called "myelin") over nerves in the brain and spinal cord.

spasticity: An unexpected increase in muscle tone or stiffness which can interfere with movement and speech and cause discomfort or pain.

steroid: Any of a group of lipids (fats) that have a certain chemical structure.

stimulants: A class of drugs that enhance the activity of monoamines (such as dopamine and norepinephrine) in the brain, increasing arousal, heart rate, blood pressure, and respiration, and decreasing appetite; includes some medications used to treat attention deficit hyperactivity disorder (e.g., methylphenidate and amphetamines), as well as cocaine and methamphetamine.

transverse myelitis (TM): A condition caused by inflammation of the spinal cord.

trigeminal neuralgia: A type of chronic pain disorder that involves sudden attacks of severe facial pain.

virus: A small organism that can infect a person and cause illness or disease.

vitamin D: A nutrient that the body needs to absorb calcium.

Glossary of Terms Related to Multiple Sclerosis

white matter: Brain tissue made up of bundles of nerve fibers (axons) covered and protected by myelin.

x-ray: A type of high-energy radiation used to diagnose diseases by making pictures of the inside of the body.

yoga: A mind and body practice that combines physical postures, breathing techniques, and meditation or relaxation.

Chapter 60 | Directory of Resources Providing Information about Multiple Sclerosis

GOVERNMENT ORGANIZATIONS

Administration for Community Living (ACL)
330 C St., S.W.
Washington, DC 20201
Toll-Free: 800-677-1116
Phone: 202-401-4634
Website: https://acl.gov
Email: aclinfo@acl.hhs.gov

Agency for Healthcare Research and Quality (AHRQ)
5600 Fishers Ln.
7th Fl.
Rockville, MD 20857
Phone: 301-427-1364
Website: www.ahrq.gov

Brain Resources and Information Network (BRAIN)
P.O. Box 5801
Bethesda, MD 20824
Toll-Free: 800-352-9424
Website: www.ninds.nih.gov/health-information/public-education/ninds-brain-educational-resources
Email: braininfo@ninds.nih.gov

Centers for Medicare & Medicaid Services (CMS)
7500 Security Blvd.
Baltimore, MD 21244
Toll-Free: 877-267-2323
Phone: 410-786-3000
TTY: 410-786-0727
Toll-Free TTY: 866-226-1819
Website: www.cms.gov

Resources here were compiled from several sources deemed reliable; all contact information was verified and updated in June 2024.

Eunice Kennedy Shriver National Institute of Child Health and Human Development (NICHD)
P.O. Box 3006
Rockville, MD 20847
Toll-Free: 800-370-2943
Phone: 301-496-5133
Website: www.nichd.nih.gov
Email: NICHDInformationResourceCenter@mail.nih.gov

Genetic and Rare Diseases Information Center (GARD)
P.O. Box 8126
Gaithersburg, MD 20898-8126
Toll-Free: 888-205-2311
Website: https://rarediseases.info.nih.gov

MyHealthfinder
1101 Wootton Pkwy., Ste. 420
Rockville, MD 20852
Website: https://health.gov/myhealthfinder
Email: healthfinder@hhs.gov

National Center for Complementary and Integrative Health (NCCIH)
9000 Rockville Pike
Bethesda, MD 20892
Toll-Free: 888-644-6226
Toll-Free TTY: 866-464-3615
Website: www.nccih.nih.gov
Email: info@nccih.nih.gov

National Eye Institute (NEI)
31 Center Dr.
MSC 2510
Bethesda, MD 20892-2510
Phone: 301-496-5248
Website: www.nei.nih.gov
Email: 2020@nei.nih.gov

National Human Genome Research Institute (NHGRI)
31 Center Dr.
MSC 2152, 9000 Rockville Pike
Bldg. 31, Rm. 4B09
Bethesda, MD 20892-2152
Phone: 301-402-0911
Fax: 301-402-2218
Website: www.genome.gov
Email: nhgripressoffice@mail.nih.gov

National Institute of Arthritis and Musculoskeletal and Skin Diseases (NIAMS)
1 AMS Cir.
Bethesda, MD 20892-3675
Toll-Free: 877-22-NIAMS (877-226-4267)
Phone: 301-495-4484
Fax: 301-718-6366
Website: www.niams.nih.gov
Email: niamsinfo@mail.nih.gov

National Institute of Diabetes and Digestive and Kidney Diseases (NIDDK)
9000 Rockville Pike
Bethesda, MD 20892
Toll-Free: 800-860-8747
Website: www.niddk.nih.gov
Email: healthinfo@niddk.nih.gov

Directory of Resources Providing Information about Multiple Sclerosis

National Institute of Environmental Health Sciences (NIEHS)
P.O. Box 12233, MD. K3-16
Research Triangle Park, NC 27709
Phone: 919-541-3345
Fax: 919-541-4395
Website: www.niehs.nih.gov
Email: webcenter@niehs.nih.gov

National Institute of Mental Health (NIMH)
6001 Executive Blvd.
MSC 9663
Bethesda, MD 20892-9663
Toll-Free: 866-615-6464
Website: www.nimh.nih.gov
Email: nimhinfo@nih.gov

National Institute of Neurological Disorders and Stroke (NINDS)
P.O. Box 5801
Bethesda, MD 20824
Toll-Free: 800-352-9424
Website: www.ninds.nih.gov

National Institutes of Health (NIH)
9000 Rockville Pike
Bethesda, MD 20892
Phone: 301-496-4000
TTY: 301-402-9612
Website: www.nih.gov
Email: olib@od.nih.gov

Office on Women's Health (OWH)
1101 Wootton Pkwy.
Rockville, MD 20852
Toll-Free: 800-994-9662
Phone: 202-690-7650

Fax: 202-205-2631
Website: www.womenshealth.gov
Email: womenshealth@hhs.gov

U.S. Department of Health and Human Services (HHS)
200 Independence Ave., S.W.
Hubert H. Humphrey Bldg.
Washington, DC 20201
Toll-Free: 877-696-6775
Website: www.hhs.gov

U.S. Department of Justice (DOJ)
950 Pennsylvania Ave., N.W.
Washington, DC 20530-0001
Phone: 202-514-2000
Toll-Free TTY: 800-877-8339
Website: www.justice.gov

U.S. Department of Veterans Affairs (VA)
810 Vermont Ave., N.W.
Washington, DC 20420
Toll-Free: 844-698-2411
Website: www.va.gov
Email: vapublicaffairs@va.gov

U.S. Equal Employment Opportunity Commission (EEOC)
131 M St., N.E.
Washington, DC 20507
Toll-Free: 800-669-4000
Toll-Free TTY: 800-669-6820
Website: www.eeoc.gov
Email: info@eeoc.gov

U.S. Food and Drug Administration (FDA)
10903 New Hampshire Ave.
Silver Spring, MD 20993-0002
Toll-Free: 888-463-6332
Website: www.fda.gov

U.S. National Library of Medicine (NLM)
8600 Rockville Pike
Bethesda, MD 20894
Toll-Free: 888-346-3656
Phone: 301-594-5983
Website: www.nlm.nih.gov
Email: NLMCommunications@nih.gov

U.S. Social Security Administration (SSA)
1100 W. High Rise
6401 Security Blvd.
Baltimore, MD 21235
Toll-Free: 800-772-1213
Toll-Free TTY: 800-325-0778
Website: www.ssa.gov

PRIVATE ORGANIZATIONS

Accelerated Cure Project (ACP)
800 Lexington St., Ste. 2
Unit 1069
Waltham, MA 02452
Phone: 781-487-0008
Website: www.acceleratedcure.org
Email: info@acceleratedcure.org

Accessible Space, Inc. (ASI)
2550 University Ave., W., Ste. 330N
St. Paul, MN 55114
Toll-Free: 800-466-7722
Phone: 651-645-7271
Toll-Free TTY: 800-627-3529
Fax: 651-645-0541
Website: www.accessiblespace.org
Email: info@accessiblespace.org

American Association of Retired Persons (AARP)
Toll-Free: 888-OUR-AARP (888-687-2277)
Phone: 202-434-3525
Toll-Free TTY: 877-434-7598
Website: www.aarp.org

American Hospital Association (AHA)
155 N. Wacker Dr.
Chicago, IL 60606
Toll-Free: 800-424-4301
Phone: 312-422-3000
Website: www.aha.org
Email: ahahelp@aha.org

The American Institute of Stress (AIS)
220 Adams Dr., Ste. 280
Unit 224
Weatherford, TX 76086
Phone: 682-239-6823
Website: www.stress.org
Email: info@stress.org

Directory of Resources Providing Information about Multiple Sclerosis

Anxiety and Depression Association of America (ADAA)
8701 Georgia Ave., Ste. 412
Silver Spring, MD 20910
Website: www.adaa.org
Email: information@adaa.org

Argentum
20 F St. N.W.
7th Fl.
Washington, DC 20001
Phone: 703-894-1805
Website: www.argentum.org
Email: info@argentum.org

Autoimmune Association
19176 Hall Rd., Ste. 130
Clinton Township, MI 48038
Phone: 586-776-3900
Fax: 586-776-3903
Website: https://autoimmune.org
Email: hello@autoimmune.org

The Consortium of Multiple Sclerosis Centers (CMSC)
3 University Plz. Dr., Ste. 116
Hackensack, NJ 07601
Phone: 201-487-1050
Fax: 862-772-7275
Website: www.mscare.org
Email: info@mscare.org

Family Caregiver Alliance® (FCA)
235 Montgomery St., Ste. 930
San Francisco, CA 94104
Toll-Free: 800-445-8106
Phone: 415-434-3388
Website: www.caregiver.org
Email: info@caregiver.org

The Foundation for Peripheral Neuropathy® (FPN)
485 E. Half Day Rd., Ste. 350
Buffalo Grove, IL 60089-8808
Toll-Free: 877-883-9942
Fax: 847-883-9960
Website: www.foundationforpn.org
Email: info@tffpn.org

International Essential Tremor Foundation (IETF)
P.O. Box 14005
Lenexa, KS 66285-4005
Toll-Free: 888-387-3667
Phone: 913-341-3880
Website: www.essentialtremor.org
Email: info@essentialtremor.org

Mental Health America (MHA)
500 Montgomery St., Ste. 820
Alexandria, VA 22314
Toll-Free: 800-969-6642
Phone: 703-684-7722
Fax: 703-684-5968
Website: www.mentalhealthamerica.net
Email: info@mhanational.org

Multiple Sclerosis Association of America (MSAA)
375 Kings Hwy., N., Ste. B
Cherry Hill, NJ 08034
Toll-Free: 800-532-7667
Fax: 856-661-9797
Website: www.mymsaa.org
Email: msaa@mymsaa.org

Multiple Sclerosis Foundation (MSF)
6520 N. Andrews Ave.
Fort Lauderdale, FL 33309-2132
Toll-Free: 888-673-6287
Phone: 954-776-6805
Fax: 954-351-0630
Website: www.msfocus.org
Email: support@msfocus.org

National Association for Continence (NAFC)
P.O. Box 1019
Charleston, SC 29402
Toll-Free: 800-252-3337
Website: www.nafc.org

National Association for Home Care & Hospice (NAHC)
228 7th St., S.E.
Washington, DC 20003
Phone: 202-547-7424
Fax: 202-547-3540
Website: www.nahc.org

National Ataxia Foundation (NAF)
600 Hwy. 169 S., Ste. 1725
Minneapolis, MN 55426
Phone: 763-553-0020
Fax: 763-553-0167
Website: www.ataxia.org
Email: naf@ataxia.org

National Center for Assisted Living (NCAL)
1201 L St., N.W.
Washington, DC 20005
Phone: 202-842-4444
Fax: 202-842-3860
Website: www.ahcancal.org
Email: ncal@ncal.org

National Center on Health, Physical Activity and Disability (NCHPAD)
3810 Ridgeway Dr.
Birmingham, AL 35209
Toll-Free: 866-866-8896
Fax: 205-975-0043
Website: www.nchpad.org
Email: nchpad@uab.edu

National Hospice and Palliative Care Organization (NHPCO)
1731 King St.
Alexandria, VA 22314
Phone: 703-837-1500
Fax: 703-837-1233
Website: www.nhpco.org

National Multiple Sclerosis Society (NMSS)
733 3rd Ave.
3rd Fl.
New York, NY 10017
Toll-Free: 800-344-4867
Website: www.nationalmssociety.org

National Organization for Rare Disorders, Inc. (NORD)
1900 Crown Colony Dr., Ste. 310
Quincy, MA 02169
Phone: 617-249-7300
Website: www.rarediseases.org

Directory of Resources Providing Information about Multiple Sclerosis

National Tay-Sachs and Allied Diseases Association (NTSAD)
2001 Beacon St., Ste. 204
Boston, MA 02135
Phone: 617-277-4463
Website: www.ntsad.org
Email: info@ntsad.org

Tremor Action Network (TAN)
P.O. Box 5013
Pleasanton, CA 94566-0513
Phone: 510-681-6565
Fax: 925-369-0485
Website: www.tremoraction.org

United Leukodystrophy Foundation (ULF)
224 N. 2nd St., Ste. 2
DeKalb, IL 60115
Toll-Free: 800-728-5483
Phone: 815-748-3211
Fax: 815-748-0844
Website: www.ulf.org
Email: office@ulf.org

Urology Care Foundation
1000 Corporate Blvd.
Linthicum, MD 21090
Toll-Free: 800-828-7866
Phone: 410-689-3700
Fax: 410-689-3800; 410-689-3998
Website: www.urologyhealth.org
Email: info@urologycarefoundation.org

Well Spouse Association (WSA)
63 W. Main St., Ste. H
Freehold, NJ 07728
Phone: 732-577-8899
Website: www.wellspouse.org
Email: info@wellspouse.org

INDEX

INDEX

Page numbers followed by "n" refer to citation information; by "t" indicate tables; and by "f" indicate figures.

A

ABA *see* Architectural Barriers Act
abnormal sensations, transverse myelitis (TM) 50
ACAA *see* Air Carrier Access Act
Accelerated Cure Project (ACP), contact information 354
Accessible Space, Inc. (ASI), contact information 354
accommodations
    disability rights laws 319
    employee with multiple sclerosis (MS) 293
acoustic neuromas, cranial nerves 13
activities of daily living (ADLs), Marburg variant multiple sclerosis (MS) 42
activity diary, described 216
activity stations, defined 266
acupuncture
    optimizing life 200
    pain 90
acute disseminated encephalomyelitis (ADEM), Marburg variant multiple sclerosis (MS) 41

ADA *see* Americans with Disabilities Act
ADA.gov
    publication
        disability rights laws 327n
Addison-Schilder disease, adrenoleukodystrophy 39
ADEM *see* acute disseminated encephalomyelitis
ADLs *see* activities of daily living
Administration for Community Living (ACL), contact information 351
adrenoleukodystrophy, Addison-Schilder disease 39
advance care planning
    overview 335–341
    social worker 313
advance directives, described 335
aerobic exercise, activity plan 214
afferent process, dendrites 6
age determination 300t
Agency for Healthcare Research and Quality (AHRQ), contact information 351
aging
    advance directive 336
    nervous system 3
AIP *see* alleged incapacitated person
Air Carrier Access Act (ACAA), defined 324

alemtuzumab
    chickenpox vaccine 260
    infusion treatment 161
    stem cell therapy 182
alleged incapacitated person (AIP),
    guardianship 331
amblyopia, exercise 168
ambulation, Marburg variant multiple
    sclerosis (MS) 41
American Association of Retired
    Persons (AARP), contact
    information 354
American Hospital
    Association (AHA), contact
    information 354
The American Institute of Stress (AIS),
    contact information 354
Americans with Disabilities
    Act (ADA), disability rights
    laws 319
anesthesia, plasmapheresis 172
anticholinergic medications, tremor 86
antidepressants, major depression 122
antiseizure medications, tremor 85
antiviral medications, transverse
    myelitis (TM) 54
Anxiety and Depression Association
    of America (ADAA), contact
    information 355
aphasia, speech and swallowing 93
arachnoid, central nervous
    system 10
Architectural Barriers Act (ABA),
    defined 327
Argentum, contact information 355
ART *see* assisted reproductive
    technology
art therapy
    defined 239
    rehabilitation medicine 195
assisted living
    described 316
    long-term care options 315

assisted reproductive
    technology (ART), pregnancy 34
assistive device, walking and
    balance 163
assistive devices
    driving considerations 284
    self-care and independence 277
    tremor 163
ataxia
    Marburg variant multiple
        sclerosis (MS) 41
    speech 93
    walking and balance 163
attention and concentration
    defined 118
    temperature sensitivity 251
Autoimmune Association, contact
    information 355
autoimmune diseases
    autoimmunity 29
    genetic susceptibility 26
    plasmapheresis 171
autologous, stem cell therapy 181
autopsy, imaging tests 149
axon
    depicted 6f
    myelin and immune system 29
    nerve tissue 6
    peripheral nervous
        system (PNS) 13
azathioprine
    neuromyelitis optica 48
    transverse myelitis (TM) 54

B

baclofen
    fatigue 77
    hyperactive bladder 113
    pain medicines 54
    sexual dysfunction 132
    spasticity 80, 163
    therapy 166

Index

bacterial infections, transverse myelitis (TM) 51
balance problems
   overview 107–109
   plaques form 66
BBB *see* blood-brain barrier
Behçet syndrome, transverse myelitis (TM) 52
benzodiazepines, tremor 86
beta-blocking drugs, tremor 85
biofeedback, pain 90
black holes, magnetic resonance imaging (MRI) 151
bladder control
   multiple sclerosis (MS) symptoms 19, 164
   Schilder disease 39
   stress management 248
blind spots, driving considerations 283
blood
   autonomic nervous system 14
   cooling vests 255
   meninges 10
   multiple sclerosis (MS) treatment 159
   nervous system 3
   plasmapheresis 171
   relapses 69
   stem cell therapy 181
   transverse myelitis (TM) 52
   vitamin D 177
blood pressure
   annual primary care evaluation 137
   autonomic nervous system 14
   intrathecal baclofen screening test 167
   plasmapheresis 174
blood tests
   neurologist 143
   transverse myelitis (TM) 52
blood-brain barrier (BBB)
   multiple sclerosis (MS) clinical relapses 71
   multiple sclerosis (MS) factors 25
blurred vision
   driving considerations 283
   plasmapheresis 174
Botox *see* botulinum toxin
botulinum toxin
   hyperactive bladder 113
   intrathecal baclofen pump 166
   spasticity 81
   tremor 86
bowel function 225
brain
   advance care planning 339
   autoimmunity 29
   bowel issues 225
   common sleep disorders 125
   depicted 9f
   described 10
   fatigue 75
   halting multiple sclerosis progression 185
   imaging tests 149
   magnetic resonance imaging (MRI) 151
   multiple sclerosis (MS) factors 25
   multiple sclerosis (MS) relapses 65
   multiple sclerosis (MS) risk 57
   music therapy 248
   natalizumab 160
   nervous system 3
   neurologist 143
   neuromyelitis optica (NMO) 46
   optic neuritis 103
   pain 89
   pediatric multiple sclerosis (MS) 61
   poor balance 107
   rehabilitation medicine 193
   Schilder disease 39
   sexual dysfunction 129
   spasticity 79, 165
   speech and swallowing 93
   transverse myelitis (TM) 49
   tremor 83
   vitamin D 178

Brain Resources and Information
  Network (BRAIN), contact
  information 351
brain scan, fatigue 75
brain stem
  central nervous system (CNS) 10
  cranial nerves 14
  evoked potentials 150
  myelin 31
brainstem syndrome, relapsing
  multiple sclerosis (MS) 143
breathing
  advance directives 336
  annual primary care evaluation 138
  autonomic nervous system 14
  exercise 240
  nervous system 4
  optimizing life 201
  pneumonia vaccine 261
  sleep apnea 126
  transverse myelitis (TM) 54
  vocal fold paralysis 100

C

caffeine
  hyperactive bladder 112
  managing bowel issues 227
  restless legs syndrome (RLS) 126
  sleep 234
  temperature sensitivity 254
  tremor 84
cardiac disease, exercise 213
cardiopulmonary resuscitation (CPR),
  advance care planning 338
CBT *see* cognitive behavioral therapy
CCRCs *see* continuing care retirement
  communities
cell body, depicted 6f
Centers for Disease Control and
  Prevention (CDC)
  publications

hepatitis B vaccine and multiple
  sclerosis 263n
insomnia 235n
keeping cool 253n
Centers for Medicare & Medicaid
  Services (CMS)
  contact information 351
  publication
    advance directives and long-
      term care 336n
central nervous system (CNS)
  bowel issues 225
  causative factors 25
  halting multiple sclerosis
    progression 185
  magnetic resonance
    imaging (MRI) 154
  Marburg variant multiple
    sclerosis (MS) 41
  neuromyelitis optica (NMO) 46
  pain 89
  pediatric multiple sclerosis (MS) 61
  relapsing multiple
    sclerosis (MS) 143
  sexual dysfunction 130, 229
  stem cell therapy 182
cerebellum
  autoimmunity 31
  brain 10
cerebral cortex
  brain 11
  autoimmunity 29
cerebral palsy (CP), spasticity 79
cerebrospinal fluid (CSF),
  neurologist 143
cerebrum, brain 10
chemotherapy
  stem cell therapy 181
  tremor 84
chickenpox
  transverse myelitis (TM) 51
  vaccine 260

Index

chiropractic care, complementary approaches 189
chronic inflammatory demyelinating polyneuropathy (CIDP)
  overview 45
  plasmapheresis 171
chronic pain
  halting multiple sclerosis (MS) progression 185
  posttraumatic stress disorder (PTSD) 240
  transverse myelitis (TM) 50
CIDP *see* chronic inflammatory demyelinating polyneuropathy
CIS *see* clinically isolated syndrome
Civil Rights of Institutionalized Persons Act (CRIPA), described 325
clinically isolated syndrome (CIS), described 144
clonus, spasticity 79
clumsiness, multiple sclerosis (MS) symptoms 19
CNS *see* central nervous system
cognitive behavioral therapy (CBT)
  insomnia 126
  multiple sclerosis (MS) symptoms 164
cognitive deficits, overview 115–119
cognitive dysfunction, multiple sclerosis (MS) symptoms 19
cognitive impairment
  accommodation 294
  cognitive deficits 116
  multiple sclerosis (MS) clinical relapses 71
  multiple sclerosis (MS) symptoms 165
  sexual dysfunction 130
  situations and solutions 297
cognitive rehabilitation therapy (CRT), rehabilitation medicine 193
cognitive-linguistic compensatory strategies, speech 94
combined dysfunction
  bladder dysfunctions 111
  defined 113
  falls 222
computed tomography (CT), transverse myelitis (TM) 52
concentration
  defined 118
  major depression 121
  Marburg variant multiple sclerosis (MS) 40
  meditation 238
  movement 247
  sleep 233
  temperature sensitivity 251
  tremor 86
connective tissue
  central nervous system (CNS) 9
  nerve tissue 5
  nervous system 3
  peripheral nervous system (PNS) 13
  transverse myelitis (TM) 52
conservatorship *see* guardianship
The Consortium of Multiple Sclerosis Centers (CMSC), contact information 355
constipation
  annual primary care evaluation 138
  bowel issues 225
  multiple sclerosis (MS) symptoms 164
  transverse myelitis (TM) 50
continuing care retirement communities (CCRCs), assisted living 316
cooling packs, temperature sensitivity 254
cooling vests, described 255
Coronavirus disease (COVID-19), described 261

corpus callosum, brain 10
cortical atrophy, myelin and immune system 30
corticosteroids
  described 20
  multiple sclerosis (MS) treatment 159
  Schilder disease 40
  tremor 84
counseling
  communication 245
  major depression 122
  multiple sclerosis (MS) symptoms 164
  pregnancy 34
  sexual dysfunction 132, 230
  social worker 312
couples counseling, communication 245
coverage requirement 300t
COVID-19 *see* Coronavirus disease
CP *see* cerebral palsy
CPR *see* cardiopulmonary resuscitation
cranial nerves
  described 13
  peripheral nervous system (PNS) 8
CRIPA *see* Civil Rights of Institutionalized Persons Act
Crohn's disease, thunder god vine 189
CRT *see* cognitive rehabilitation therapy
CSF *see* cerebrospinal fluid
CSF *see* cerebrospinal fluid
CT *see* computed tomography

D

DBS *see* deep brain stimulation
deep brain stimulation (DBS)
  multiple sclerosis (MS) symptoms 163
  surgery 86

dementia
  exercise and movement 168
  guardianship 331
  long-term care 315
  Schilder disease 39
dendrites
  defined 6
  depicted 6f
  peripheral nervous system (PNS) 13
depression
  annual primary care evaluation 138
  building resilience 204
  exercise and movement 168
  fatigue 76
  halting multiple sclerosis progression 185
  insomnia 125
  Marburg variant multiple sclerosis (MS) 40
  meditation 238
  multiple sclerosis (MS) symptoms 19, 164
  optimizing life 200
  overview 121–123
  pain 90
  posttraumatic stress disorder (PTSD) 239
  sexual dysfunction 130, 229
  transverse myelitis (TM) 50
developmental disorders, rehabilitation 193
diabetes
  annual primary care evaluation 137
  diet 209
  exercise 213
  fatigue 76
  hepatitis B vaccine 263
  sexual dysfunction 130
  tremor 84
dialysis
  advance directives 336
  plasmapheresis 171

Index

diarrhea
  bowel issues 226
  oral treatments 161
  thunder god vine 190
diencephalon, brain 10
diet changes
  diet 209
  fatigue 76
  managing bowel issues 226
diffusion-tensor magnetic resonance imaging (DT-MRI), Marburg variant multiple sclerosis (MS) 41
disabilities
  disability rights laws 319
  Kurtzke Disability Status Scale (DSS) 154
  long-term rehabilitation 54
  rehabilitation medicine 194
  tremor 83
  work 307
disability
  cognitive deficits 116
  diet 207
  exercise 218
  falls 222
  fatigue 75
  inheritance 23
  laws 319
  Marburg variant multiple sclerosis (MS) 19
  multiple sclerosis (MS) relapses 65
  neuromyelitis optica (NMO) 48
  overview 299–309
  pain 89
  posttraumatic stress disorder (PTSD) 239
  rehabilitation 142, 193
  restless legs syndrome (RLS) 126
  sexual dysfunction 130
  smoking 62
disability benefits, overview 299–309

discomfort
  multiple sclerosis (MS) relapse 69
  optic neuritis 103
  plasmapheresis 172
  stress management 248
  transverse myelitis (TM) 50
disease modifying treatments (DMTs), pregnancy 34
disease-modifying therapy
  diet 209
  infusion treatment 160
  multiple sclerosis (MS) clinical relapses 70
  plasmapheresis 174
dizziness
  Marburg variant multiple sclerosis (MS) 41
  multiple sclerosis (MS) symptoms 19
  plasmapheresis 174
  spasticity 166
DMTs *see* disease modifying treatments
DNH *see* do not hospitalize
DNI *see* do not intubate
DNR *see* do not resuscitate
do not hospitalize (DNH), advance care planning 338
do not intubate (DNI), advance care planning 338
do not resuscitate (DNR), advance care planning 338
dopaminergic medications, tremor 86
double vision
  delay future attacks 58
  driving 283
  multiple sclerosis (MS) relapses 66
  multiple sclerosis (MS) symptoms 19, 163
DT-MRI *see* diffusion-tensor magnetic resonance imaging
durable power of attorney for health care, advance directives 335

dysarthria
    Schilder disease 39
    speech 93
dystonia
    speech 93
    tremor 86

E

EBV *see* Epstein-Barr virus
eculizumab, neuromyelitis
    optica (NMO) 48
EDSS *see* Kurtzke Expanded Disability
    Status Scale
Education for All Handicapped
    Children Act *see* Individuals with
    Disabilities Education Act
electromyogram 85
endocrine function,
    meditation 238
endoneurium 13
epineurium 13
epithalamus 11
Epstein-Barr virus (EBV)
    infection 26
    multiple sclerosis 22, 59
Eunice Kennedy Shriver National
    Institute of Child Health and
    Human Development (NICHD)
    contact information 352
    publications
        nervous system 4n, 15n
        parts of nervous system 5n
        rehabilitation medicine 195n
evoked potentials, described 149
exacerbation (relapse)
    described 20
    driving 283
    exercise 169
    myelin and immune system 30
    neurologist 141
executive functions, described 118

exercise
    diet 210
    fatigue 75
    guidelines overview 213–219
    hyperactive bladder 112
    imbalance 108
    neurologist 141
    pain 90
    rehabilitation 194
    resilience 204
    speech 94
    tremors 87
    vocal fold paralysis 100

F

Fair Housing Act, described 323
falls
    bladder dysfunction link 221–223
    imbalance 107
    mobility challenges 268
Family Caregiver Alliance® (FCA),
    contact information 355
family history 58
fasciculus 13
fasting, described 208
fatigue
    accommodation 294
    budget approach 265
    chronic inflammatory
        demyelinating polyneuropathy
        (CIDP) 45
    cognitive function 116
    diet 207
    driving 283
    exercise 168, 213, 219
    imbalance 107
    insomnia 125
    intrathecal baclofen 166
    major depression 122
    meditation 238
    multiple sclerosis (MS)
        specialist 138

Index

fatigue, *continued*
   neurologist 141
   overview 75–77
   pain 90
   plasmapheresis 174
   power mobility 277
   pregnancy 33
   relapsing multiple sclerosis (MS) 143
   resilience 204
   restless legs syndrome (RLS) 127
   sexual dysfunction 129, 229
   sleep 125
   sleep apnea 126
   spasticity 163
   speaking 97
   swallowing 96
   temperature sensitivity 255
   tremors 84
fine motor impairment, accommodation 295
fingolimod 161, 259
Flu Mist 259
flu vaccine *see* influenza
focused ultrasound, tremors 86
The Foundation for Peripheral Neuropathy® (FPN), contact information 355
functional system (FS) scores 155t
fungal infections, transverse myelitis (TM) 51

G

gabapentin
   pain 54
   fatigue 77, 164
   spasticity 163, 166
gait
   imbalance 108
   Marburg variant or malignant multiple sclerosis (MS) 41
   music therapy 247
ganglia 3, 8
Gardasil-9, human papillomavirus (HPV) vaccination 261
GBS *see* Guillain-Barré syndrome
general intelligence, described 119
Genetic and Rare Diseases Information Center (GARD)
   contact information 352
   publication
      Alzheimer disease and home safety 275n
      pediatric multiple sclerosis 61n
Goodpasture syndrome, plasmapheresis 171
gross motor impairment, accommodation 295
guardianship, overview 329–333
Guillain-Barré syndrome (GBS)
   chronic inflammatory demyelinating polyneuropathy (CIDP) 45
   plasmapheresis 171

H

HDIT *see* high-dose immunosuppressive therapy
hearing loss
   evoked potentials 150
   Marburg variant or malignant multiple sclerosis (MS) 41
heartbeat, plasmapheresis 174
heat sensitivity, accommodation 295
hepatitis B (HepB)
   vaccine 262
   viral infection 51
HepB *see* hepatitis B
HIV *see* human immunodeficiency virus
HLA-DRB1 22

home accessibility features,
    overview 271–275
homeostasis
    marburg variant multiple
        sclerosis (MS) 41
    nervous system 3
    pain 89
    pediatric multiple sclerosis (MS) 61
    relapsing multiple
        sclerosis (MS) 143
    sexual dysfunction 130
    stem cell therapy 182, 229
    transverse myelitis (TM) 51
HPV *see* human papillomavirus
human immunodeficiency
    virus (HIV), plasmapheresis 172
human papillomavirus (HPV)
    vaccine 261
hyperactive bladder, described 112
hypnosis, pain 90
hypoactive bladder, described 112
hypothalamus 10

I

ibuprofen, pain 54, 90
IDEA *see* Individuals with Disabilities
    Education Act
IgG *see* immunoglobulin G
IL-7R 22
imbalance
    overview 107–109
    see also poor balance
immune system
    chronic inflammatory
        demyelinating polyneuropathy
        (CIDP) 46
    corticosteroids 159
    diet 207
    multiple sclerosis (MS) 29, 57, 185
    multiple sclerosis (MS) relapse 66
    myelin 29

natalizumab 160
neuromyelitis optica (NMO) 47
plasmapheresis 171
shingles 260
sleep 125
stem cell therapy 181
transverse myelitis (TM) 50
vitamin D therapy 177
immunoglobulin G (IgG), multiple
    sclerosis (MS) 143
immunosuppressive drugs,
    neuromyelitis optica (NMO) 48
immunosuppressive therapy, Schilder
    disease 40
impaired sensorimotor function,
    driving 283
incontinence
    bladder dysfunction 111, 221
    bowel issues 226
    multiple sclerosis (MS)
        specialist 138
    transverse myelitis (TM) 50
Individuals with Disabilities Education
    Act (IDEA)
inebilizumab, neuromyelitis
    optica (NMO) 48
inflammation
    blindness 162
    children 61
    clinically isolated
        syndrome (CIS) 145
    corticosteroids 159
    fatigue 75
    Marburg variant or malignant
        multiple sclerosis (MS) 40
    neuromyelitis optica (NMO) 46
    optic neuritis 103
    posttraumatic stress
        disorder (PTSD) 239
    steroid relapses 66
    transverse myelitis (TM) 49
    Wahls protocol 208

Index

influenza (flu) vaccine 259
information processing
   described 117
   Marburg variant or malignant multiple sclerosis (MS) 40
   multiple sclerosis (MS) 115
   speech 94
inheritance
   multiple sclerosis (MS) 23
   neuromyelitis optica (NMO) 48
insomnia
   described 125
   major depression 122
interferon beta, Schilder disease 40
intermittent pain 89
International Essential Tremor Foundation (IETF), contact information 355
intrathecal baclofen (ITB), spasticity 80, 165
intrauterine devices (IUDs) 35
intravenous methylprednisolone (IVMP) 21, 66
involuntary nervous system 9
Island of Reil 10
ITB *see* intrathecal baclofen
IUDs *see* intrauterine devices
IVMP *see* intravenous methylprednisolone

J

jogging, exercise 213, 240
joint swelling, thunder god vine 190

K

ketogenic diet, described 209
Kurtzke Expanded Disability Status Scale (EDSS) 155t

L

Lambert-Eaton syndrome, plasmapheresis 171
LARCs *see* long-acting reversible contraceptives
laryngeal electromyography, vocal fold paralysis 100
lesions
   cardio workouts 219
   clinically isolated syndrome (CIS) 144
   fatigue 75
   Marburg variant or malignant multiple sclerosis (MS) 40
   multiple sclerosis (MS) 17, 186
   myelin and immune system 30
   ocrelizumab 161
   optic neuritis 104
   pain 89
   posttraumatic stress disorder (PTSD) 239
   Schilder disease 39
   sexual dysfunction 130
   smoking 27
   speech and swallowing 93
   transverse myelitis (TM) 52
   tremors 87
   vitamin D 178
lifestyle changes
   diet 209
   fatigue 77
   tremors 87
living will, advance directives 335
long-acting reversible contraceptives (LARCs), pregnancy 35
long-term care services 315
low blood pressure
   intrathecal baclofen (ITB) pump 168
   plasmapheresis 174
low thyroid hormone, fatigue 75

lower back pain, transverse
    myelitis (TM) 50
lumbar puncture
    described 149
    intrathecal baclofen (ITB)
        pump 167
    neurologist 141
    transverse myelitis (TM) 53
lupus *see* systemic lupus erythematosus

M

magnetic resonance imaging (MRI)
    acoustic neuromas 14
    focused ultrasound 86
    Marburg variant or malignant
        multiple sclerosis (MS) 41
    optic neuritis 104
    overview 151–154
    postpartum 35
    transverse myelitis (TM) 52
    vitamin D therapy 178
malignant multiple sclerosis *see*
    Marburg variant
Marburg variant (malignant) multiple
    sclerosis (MS), overview 40–42
Medicare
    advance care planning 339
    continuing care retirement
        communities (CCRCs) 317
    disability benefits 307
medications
    assisted living 316
    depression 122, 165
    disease-modifying treatments 160
    eye and vision 163
    fatigue 76, 277
    hyperactive bladder 113
    hypoactive bladder 112
    imbalance 108
    insomnia 125
    intrathecal baclofen (ITB)
        pump 167

managing bowel issues 225
neuromyelitis optica (NMO) 48
pain 90
plasmapheresis 171
restless legs syndrome (RLS) 127
sexual
    dysfunction 130, 132, 164, 230
sleep 233
spasticity 80, 163, 166
speech 95
stem cell therapy 181
stress 237
temperature sensitivity 251
transverse myelitis (TM) 53
tremors 84
urinary incontinence 223
meditation
    described 237
    pain 90
    posttraumatic stress
        disorder (PTSD) 239
MedlinePlus
    publications
        multiple sclerosis 17n, 23n
        neuromyelitis optica 48n
        NIH study for severe multiple
            sclerosis 58n
memory
    accommodation 294
    cognitive rehabilitation
        therapy (CRT) 193
    depression 122
    driving 283
    general intelligence 119
    Marburg variant or malignant
        multiple sclerosis (MS) 40
    music therapy 247
    rehabilitative/assistive
        technology 194
    sleep 233
    sleep apnea 126
meninges
    depicted 9f
    described 10

Index

meningiomas 10
Mental Health America (MHA), contact information 355
methylphenidate
    imbalance 108
    fatigue 164
methylprednisolone
    multiple sclerosis (MS) exacerbation 21
    multiple sclerosis (MS) 159
    optic neuritis 104
    pregnancy 34
    steroid relapses 66
    transverse myelitis (TM) 53
MFS *see* Miller-Fisher syndrome
MG *see* myasthenia gravis
Miller-Fisher syndrome (MFS), plasmapheresis 171
mindfulness
    described 240
    multiple sclerosis (MS) 201
    resilience 205
mobility aid
    fatigue/weakness 294
    mobility challenges 267
    rehabilitative/assistive technology 194
mobility challenges, overview 265–269
mood changes, multiple sclerosis (MS) 19, 200
Morton neuroma 7
motor impulses 8, 12
MRI *see* magnetic resonance imaging
Multiple Sclerosis Association of America (MSAA), contact information 355
Multiple Sclerosis Foundation (MSF), contact information 356
muscle spasms
    early multiple sclerosis (MS) 19
    insomnia 125
    neuromyelitis optica (NMO) 48
    spasticity 79
    speech 94
    transverse myelitis (TM) 50
muscle stiffness
    early multiple sclerosis (MS) 19
    intrathecal baclofen (ITB) pump 165
muscle stretching 218
muscle weakness
    driving 283
    multiple sclerosis (MS) 19, 163, 277
    neuromyelitis optica (NMO) 48
    sexual dysfunction 130, 229
    temperature sensitivity 251
music therapy, overview 247–249
myasthenia gravis (MG), neuromyelitis optica (NMO) 46
mycophenolate mofetil, transverse myelitis (TM) 54
myelin
    children 61
    eye and vision 162
    immune system 29
    pain 89
    stem cell therapy 181
    temperature sensitivity 251
    transverse myelitis (TM) 49
myelin sheath, depicted 6f, 18f, 30f
myelinoclastic diffuse sclerosis *see* Schilder disease
MyHealthfinder, contact information 352

N

narcotics, pain 91
natalizumab, infusion treatment 160
National Association for Continence (NAFC), contact information 356
National Association for Home Care & Hospice (NAHC), contact information 356

National Ataxia Foundation (NAF), contact information 356
National Center for Assisted Living (NCAL), contact information 356
National Center for Complementary and Integrative Health (NCCIH) contact information 352
    publication
        thunder god vine 191n
National Center on Health, Physical Activity and Disability (NCHPAD), contact information 356
National Council on Disability (NCD) publication
        guardianship 333n
National Eye Institute (NEI), contact information 352
National Hospice and Palliative Care Organization (NHPCO), contact information 356
National Human Genome Research Institute (NHGRI), contact information 352
National Institute of Arthritis and Musculoskeletal and Skin Diseases (NIAMS) contact information 352
    publication
        autoimmune diseases 29n
National Institute of Diabetes and Digestive and Kidney Diseases (NIDDK), contact information 352
National Institute of Environmental Health Sciences (NIEHS), contact information 353
National Institute of Mental Health (NIMH) contact information 353
    publication
        chronic illness and mental health 123n

National Institute of Neurological Disorders and Stroke (NINDS) contact information 353
    publications
        chronic inflammatory demyelinating polyneuropathy (CIDP) 46n
        multiple sclerosis 20n, 23n, 27n, 31n, 65n, 70n, 71n, 132n, 165n
        neurological diagnostic tests and procedures 150n
        neuromyelitis optica 49n
        Schilder disease 40n
        transverse myelitis (TM) 55n
        tremors 87n
National Institute on Aging (NIA) publications
    advance care planning 336n, 341n
    long-term care facilities 317n
National Institute on Deafness and Other Communication Disorders (NIDCD) publication
    vocal fold paralysis 101n
National Institutes of Health (NIH) publications
    immune system 186n
    stem cell transplant 183n
    vitamin D levels 187n
National Institutes of Health (NIH), contact information 353
National Multiple Sclerosis Society (NMSS), contact information 356
National Organization for Rare Disorders, Inc. (NORD), contact information 356
National Tay-Sachs and Allied Diseases Association (NTSAD), contact information 357

Index

National Voter Registration
    Act (NVRA), described 324
nerve cell, depicted 18f
nerve fiber, depicted 18f
nerve tissue, described 5
nervous system
    bowel issues 225
    children 61
    magnetic resonance
        imaging (MRI) 154
    Marburg variant or malignant
        multiple sclerosis (MS) 41
    multiple sclerosis (MS) 17, 25, 185
    neuromyelitis optica (NMO) 46
    overview 3–15
    pain 89
    relapsing multiple
        sclerosis (MS) 143
    sexual dysfunction 130
    sexual dysfunction 229
    stem cell therapy 182
    transverse myelitis (TM) 51
    Wahls protocol 208
nucleus, depicted 6f
neurogenic pain 89
neuroglia, described 7
neuro-inflammation, clinical
    relapses 68
neurological disorder
    diagnostic tests 149
    hepatitis B (HepB) vaccine 263
    tremors 84
neurologist
    depression 122
    magnetic resonance
        imaging (MRI) 151
    multiple sclerosis (MS) 162
    optic neuritis 104
    overview 141–145
    pregnancy 34
    temperature sensitivity 257
neuromyelitis optica (NMO)
    overview 46–49
    transverse myelitis (TM) 50

neuron
    described 5
    depicted 6f
    fatigue 75
neurotoxins, tremors 84
neurotransmitters, glia 5
NIH News in Health
    publications
        managing multiple sclerosis 59n
        multiple sclerosis 29n, 31n
NMO *see* neuromyelitis optica
node of Ranvier, depicted 6f
numbness
    clinical relapses 68
    early multiple sclerosis (MS)
        symptoms 19
    exercise 214
    falls 223
    Marburg variant or malignant
        multiple sclerosis (MS) 41
    sexual dysfunction 130
    transverse myelitis (TM) 50
nursing homes, described 316
NVRA *see* National Voter Registration
    Act

O

obesity
    children 62
    diet 207
    sexual dysfunction 130
occupational therapy
    fatigue 164
    intrathecal baclofen (ITB)
        pump 167
    rehabilitation medicine 193
    tremors 87
ocrelizumab 161, 182
Office of Disability Employment
    Policy (ODEP)
    publication
        accommodation 297n

Office on Women's Health (OWH), contact information 353
ONTT *see* Optic Neuritis Treatment Trial
opioids, pain 91
optic neuritis
    clinically isolated syndrome (CIS) 144
    multiple sclerosis (MS) 19, 162
    neuromyelitis optica (NMO) 46
    overview 103–105
    relapsing multiple sclerosis (MS) 143
    steroid relapses 66
Optic Neuritis Treatment Trial (ONTT), steroid relapses 66
OTC *see* over-the-counter
otolaryngologist, vocal fold paralysis 100
over-the-counter (OTC)
    managing bowel issues 227
    pain 90
    sleep 235
overheating, described 215
oxybutynin, hyperactive bladder 113

P

pain
    driving 283
    early multiple sclerosis (MS) symptoms 19
    fatigue 75
    insomnia 125
    intrathecal baclofen (ITB) pump 165
    major depression 122
    meditation 238
    mindfulness 240
    multiple sclerosis (MS) 164, 185
    multiple sclerosis (MS) relapse 69
    music therapy 248
    neuromyelitis optica (NMO) 46
    optic neuritis 103
    overview 89–91
    plasmapheresis 172
    resilience 204
    sexual dysfunction 130
    Shingles 260
    spasticity 163
    transverse myelitis (TM) 50
paralysis
    multiple sclerosis (MS) 20, 57
    neuromyelitis optica (NMO) 48
    transverse myelitis (TM) 50
    see also vocal fold paralysis
paraparesis, transverse myelitis (TM) 50
paraplegia, transverse myelitis (TM) 50
pediatric multiple sclerosis (MS), overview 61–63
perception 118
perineurium 13
peripheral nervous system (PNS), described 12
pets, coping with stress 240
physical exam
    fatigue 75
    plasmapheresis 172
    tremors 84
physical therapy
    chronic inflammatory demyelinating polyneuropathy (CIDP) 46
    fatigue 76
    pain 90, 164
    pregnancy 34
    rehabilitation medicine 194
    spasticity 163
physiology, meditation 238
Pilates 218

Index

plaque
    clinical relapses 69
    intrathecal baclofen (ITB)
        pump 165
    Marburg variant or malignant
        multiple sclerosis (MS) 40
    multiple sclerosis (MS) relapses 65
    myelin and immune system 30
    optic neuritis 104
plasma exchange
plasma exchange *see* plasmapheresis
plasmapheresis
    neuromyelitis optica (NMO) 48
    overview 171–175
    transverse myelitis (TM) 53
pneumonia
    swallowing 95
    transverse myelitis (TM) 51
    vaccine 260
Pneumovax 23, pneumonia
    vaccine 260
PNS *see* peripheral nervous system
poor balance, overview 107–109
posttraumatic stress
    disorder (PTSD),
    overview 239–241
power mobility, overview 279–281
pregnancy, overview 33–35
Prevnar 13, pneumonia vaccine 260
primary care evaluation,
    overview 137–139
primary-progressive multiple
    sclerosis (MS)
    clinical relapses 68
    described 19
    ocrelizumab 160
progressive-relapsing multiple
    sclerosis (MS), described 19
pseudobulbar affect 165
psoriasis, pregnancy 33
psychiatric problems, posttraumatic
    stress disorder (PTSD) 239

psychotherapy
    fatigue 164
    support network 312
PTSD *see* posttraumatic stress disorder

Q

QOL *see* quality of life
quality of life (QOL)
    cardio workouts 219
    cognitive problems 119
    depression 121
    fatigue 75
    meditation 238
    multiple sclerosis (MS) 139
    neurologist 141
    optic neuritis 103
    pain 91
    rehabilitation medicine 195
    resilience 204
    restless legs syndrome (RLS) 127
    sexual dysfunction 130, 229
    swallowing problems 93
    transverse myelitis (TM) 55

R

RA *see* rheumatoid arthritis
radiofrequency ablation, surgery 86
radiographic relapses, multiple
    sclerosis (MS) 66
radiologist 145, 154
range of motion exercises 218
rapid eye movement (REM),
    sleep 233
recovery
    corticosteroids 159
    driving 284
    multiple sclerosis (MS) 23, 65
    neuromyelitis optica (NMO) 47
    optic neuritis 103
    transverse myelitis (TM) 49

recreational therapy, multiple
sclerosis (MS) 194
rehabilitation
  multiple sclerosis (MS)
    relapses 21, 71
  nervous system 3
  neuromyelitis
    optica (NMO) 49
  Social Security disability
    benefits 307
  transverse myelitis (TM) 54
Rehabilitation Act,
  described 326
relapse *see* exacerbation
relapsing-remitting MS (RRMS)
  stem cell therapy 182
  mitoxantrone 161
  ketogenic diet 209
  described 17
  clinical relapses 68
relaxation
  clinical relapses 70
  fatigue 164
  meditation 238
  mindfulness 240
  pain 90
  rehabilitation medicine 194
  resilience 205
  spasticity 165
  speech 94
REM *see* rapid eye movement
resilience, overview 203–206
restless legs syndrome (RLS),
  described 126
rheumatoid arthritis (RA)
  genetic susceptibility 26
  pregnancy 33
rituximab
  neuromyelitis optica (NMO) 48
  transverse myelitis (TM) 54
RLS *see* restless legs syndrome
RRMS *see* relapsing-remitting MS

S

satralizumab, neuromyelitis
  optica (NMO) 48
Schilder disease, overview 39–40
Schwann cell
  depicted 6f
  nerve tissue 7
SCI *see* spinal cord injury
scleroderma, transverse
  myelitis (TM) 52
secondary progressive
  defined 144
  plasma exchange 159
selective serotonin reuptake
  inhibitors (SSRIs), insomnia 125
self-advocacy, overview 287–289
sensory impulses, brain 11
sensory input, nervous system 4
sexual concerns, sexual
  dysfunction 133
sexual dysfunction
  multiple sclerosis (MS)
    symptoms 164
  overview 129–133, 229
  pregnancy 34
  transverse myelitis (TM) 50
shingles
  transverse myelitis (TM) 51
  vaccine 260
Shingrix vaccine, described 260
sildenafil, sexual dysfunction 230
Sjögren syndrome (SS), neuromyelitis
  optica (NMO) 46
skin infections
  multiple sclerosis (MS) relapse 69
  transverse myelitis (TM) 51
skull, depicted 9f
SLE *see* systemic lupus erythematosus
sleep apnea
  defined 126
  fatigue 76
  sleep disorders 125

Index

sleep patterns, complementary approach 189
SLP *see* speech and language pathologist
smoking
  cause of multiple sclerosis (MS) 22
  optimizing life 199
  pediatric multiple sclerosis (MS) 62
  sexual dysfunction 130
Social Security, disability benefits 299
Social Security Disability Insurance (SSDI), disability benefits 299
social stress, posttraumatic stress disorder (PTSD) 239
social worker
  general intelligence 119
  pets 241
  support networks 311
Solu-Medrol®, optic neuritis 104
somatic nervous system, peripheral nervous system (PNS) 8
spasticity
  annual primary care evaluation 138
  described 165
  exercise 218
  fatigue 75
  Marburg variant multiple sclerosis (MS) 41
  multiple sclerosis (MS) symptoms overview 79–81
  sexual dysfunction 130, 229
speaking
  described 97
  rehabilitation medicine 193
  vocal fold paralysis 100
speech and language pathologist (SLP) 94
speech and language therapy, described 194
speech disorder 93
speech patterns 94
speech techniques 94
spinal cord injury (SCI)
  evoked potentials 149
  multiple sclerosis (MS) specialist 137
  rehabilitative/assistive technology 194
  spasticity 79
spirituality 205
SS *see* Sjögren syndrome
SSDI *see* Social Security Disability Insurance
SSI *see* Supplemental Security Income
SSRI *see* selective serotonin reuptake inhibitor
SSRIs *see* selective serotonin reuptake inhibitors
steady pain, described 89
stem cell therapy, overview 181–183
stomach pain, multiple sclerosis (MS) relapse 69
stress
  coping with 237, 248
  driving 284
  fatigue 164
  multiple sclerosis (MS) relapse 69
  nervous system 3
  sleep 125
  transverse myelitis (TM) 50
  tremors 83
suicide, depression 121
Supplemental Security Income (SSI), disability benefits 299
support networks, overview 311–313
Surveillance, Epidemiology, and End Results (SEER) Program publications
  nervous system 3n, 15n
swallowing dysfunction 95
Swank diet, described 207

swelling
	glatiramer acetate 160
	hypoactive bladder 112
	plasmapheresis 171
	transverse myelitis (TM) 53
swimming
	fatigue 77, 213
	multiple sclerosis (MS) 218
	posttraumatic stress
		disorder (PTSD) 240
	temperature sensitivity 252
systemic lupus erythematosus (SLE)
	transverse myelitis (TM) 51
	neuromyelitis optica (NMO) 46

T

tadalafil, sexual dysfunction 230
tai chi
	complementary approach 218
	imbalance 108
	pain management 90
	posttraumatic stress disorder
		(PTSD) 240
TBI *see* traumatic brain injury
TCM *see* traditional Chinese medicine
Telecommunications Act,
	described 322
telehealth 71
temperature sensitivity,
	overview 251–257
tenderness, thunder god vine 190
thalamus
	deep brain stimulation (DBS) 86
	described 10
thyroid disorder, tremors 84
tingling
	chronic inflammatory
		demyelinating
			polyneuropathy (CIDP) 45
	clinical relapses 68
	exercise 214

intrathecal baclofen (ITB) 168
	multiple sclerosis (MS) 19, 185
	pain 89
	transverse myelitis (TM) 50
tiredness
	multiple sclerosis (MS) 163
	sleep apnea 126
tizanidine
	fatigue 77
	spasticity 80, 166
	transverse myelitis (TM) 54
TM *see* transverse myelitis
tolterodine, hyperactive bladder 113
tracheotomy, vocal fold paralysis 101
traditional Chinese medicine (TCM),
	multiple sclerosis (MS) 189
tranquilizers *see* benzodiazepines
transverse myelitis (TM)
	overview 49–55
	relapsing multiple sclerosis
		(MS) 143
	traumatic brain injury (TBI),
		spasticity 79
Tremor Action Network (TAN),
	contact information 357
tremors
	Marburg variant or malignant
		multiple sclerosis (MS) 41
	multiple sclerosis (MS) 163
	overview 83–87
	sexual dysfunction 130
	speech 94
trigeminal neuralgia, pain 20, 90, 164
tumors, vocal fold paralysis 99
type 1 diabetes 26

U

U.S. Department of Health &
	Human Services (HHS), contact
	information 353
U.S. Department of Justice (DOJ),
	contact information 353

Index

U.S. Department of Veterans Affairs (VA)
contact information 353
publications
activities and exercise
program 217n
avoiding falls 108n, 109n
bladder changes in multiple
sclerosis 113n
bowel management in multiple
sclerosis 227n
children and multiple sclerosis
risk 63n
common sleep disorders and
multiple sclerosis 127n
complementary therapies and
multiple sclerosis 189n
coping strategies for people
with multiple sclerosis 241n
depression 123n
diagnosing multiple sclerosis
using the McDonald
criteria 145n, 154n
dietary changes and multiple
sclerosis 210n
driving 285n
exercise tips for multiple
sclerosis 219n
falls in multiple sclerosis
bladder problems 223n
Kurtzke Expanded Disability
Status Scale 157n
living multiple sclerosis 201n
magnetic resonance
imaging (MRI) 153n
managing spasticity with
an intrathecal baclofen
pump 168n
mobility challenges 269n
multiple sclerosis 91n, 108n,
142n, 169n
multiple sclerosis and bladder
issues 221n, 222n
multiple sclerosis and
cognition 119n
multiple sclerosis and
fatigue 77n
multiple sclerosis and heat
tolerance 252n, 257n
multiple sclerosis and office
visit 139n
multiple sclerosis
relapses 21n, 66n, 67n
music therapy in multiple
sclerosis 249n
optic neuritis 105n
power mobility 280n, 281n
pregnancy in multiple
sclerosis 35n
relationships 245n
resilience 206n
scooter or power
wheelchair 280n
self-advocacy 289n
sexual dysfunction and multiple
sclerosis 130n, 131n, 133n,
231n
social worker support for
veterans and
families 313n
spasticity 81n
speech and swallowing 96n
stem cell therapy for multiple
sclerosis 182n
stress and multiple
sclerosis 239n
swallowing, speaking, and
thinking 97n, 115n
tips for good sleep 234n
vaccines and multiple
sclerosis 262n
vitamin D 179n
U.S. Equal Employment Opportunity
Commission (EEOC), contact
information 353

U.S. Food and Drug
    Administration (FDA), contact
    information 354
U.S. National Library of
    Medicine (NLM), contact
    information 354
U.S. Social Security
    Administration (SSA)
    contact information 354
    publications
        disability benefits 309n
        malignant multiple sclerosis 42n
United Leukodystrophy
    Foundation (ULF), contact
    information 357
urinary discomfort 69
Urology Care Foundation, contact
    information 357

V

vaccinations, overview 259–263
VAEHA *see* Voting Accessibility for the
    Elderly and Handicapped Act
vardenafil, sexual dysfunction 230
varicella zoster
    transverse myelitis (TM) 51
    vaccine 259
vascular disorders
    sleep apnea 126
    transverse myelitis (TM) 52
VCR *see* vestibulo-collic reflex
verbal fluency, described 118
vestibulocochlear nerve 14
vestibulo-collic reflex (VCR), visual
    perceptual skills 118
viral infections
    infusion treatment 160
    transverse myelitis (TM) 51
visceral efferent nervous system 9
vision problems
    multiple sclerosis (MS) 19, 162
    optic neuritis 103

visual perceptual skills, described 118
vitamin D
    children 62
    multiple sclerosis (MS) 22, 59, 186
    pregnancy 35
vitamin D therapy,
    overview 177–179
vocal cord paralysis *see* vocal fold
    paralysis
vocal fold paralysis,
    overview 99–101
vocational rehabilitation, multiple
    sclerosis (MS) 195
voluntary nervous system 9
Voting Accessibility for the Elderly
    and Handicapped Act (VAEHA),
    described 324

W

Wahls protocol, described 208
walker
    imbalance 108, 163
    Marburg variant or malignant
        multiple sclerosis (MS) 41
    mobility challenges 265
    neurologist 141
    rehabilitative/assistive
        technology 194
    self-care 277
Well Spouse Association (WSA),
    contact information 357
wellness
    advance care planning 339
    multiple sclerosis
        (MS) 189, 199, 287
wheelchairs
    aerobic workout 219
    body temperature 252
    driving safety 284
    Fair Housing Act 323
    Kurtzke Disability Status Scale
        (DSS) 156t

Index

wheelchairs, *continued*
    Marburg variant or malignant multiple sclerosis (MS) 41
    neurologist 142
    pneumonia 261
    rehabilitative/assistive technology 194
    self-care 277
    transverse myelitis (TM) 50
    see also power mobility
white matter
    Marburg variant or malignant multiple sclerosis (MS) 41
    multiple sclerosis (MS) 29
work incentives, Social Security 307
workplace
    accommodation 294
    occupational therapy 193

Y

yoga
    complementary approach 218
    pain management 90
    physical wellness 199, 201
    posttraumatic stress disorder (PTSD) 240
    spasticity 162